BREAST CANCER HELP GUIDE

Lightening the Burden of Your Journey through Breast Cancer

Diagnosis and Treatment

By: Dr. Chris Charlton

Breast Cancer Help Center

305 Spring Creek Village, Ste 425
Dallas, Texas 75248
www.BreastCancerHelpCenter.org

DISCLAIMER

This publication is intended to provide helpful and informative material. It is
not intended to diagnose, treat, cure, or prevent any health problem or
condition, nor is intended to replace the advice of a physician. No action
should be taken solely on the contents of this book. Always consult your
physician or qualified health-care professional on any matters regarding your
health and before adopting any suggestions in this book or drawing
inferences from it.

The author and publisher specifically disclaim all responsibility for any
liability, loss or risk, personal or otherwise, which is incurred as a
consequence, directly or indirectly, from the use or application of any
contents of this book. Any and all product names referenced within this book
are the trademarks of their respective owners. None of these owners have
sponsored, authorized, endorsed, or approved this book.

Always read all information provided by the manufacturers' product labels
before using their products. The author and publisher are not responsible for
claims made by manufacturers.

This book is dedicated to all the men and women, who have suffered, are suffering and have yet to suffer from breast cancer. I solemnly express my gratitude to all my patients who have chosen to face breast cancer head on with hope and optimism. Not only has your courage humbled me but it has allowed me to better myself in this field as well. I hope this book will serve its purpose of guiding and helping all of those diagnosed with breast cancer.

My thanks and my prayers go out to you all.

A Message to Breast Cancer Victims and Their Families

Breast Cancer, for a long time now, has been thought by many as an "incurable" disease. While this kind of thinking may still hold some truth to it, the reality of the situation is that breast cancer —given the precise amount of preparation, information, guidance and early detection— is indeed curable! I am Dr. Chris Charlton. My life's work has been devoted to years of practice with the purpose of understanding this horrible disease in the pursuit of treatment, research and, most of all, giving hope to those who have suffered in its grip, families and victims alike.

The content of this book is not, in any way, meant to substitute medical advice. Consulting with your physician is critical to getting treatment. This book, however, in all its purposes may act as a reference with which you can gather useful information and thus, educate yourself or your loved ones with regards to the plight of having breast cancer. More importantly, this book is meant to "ease your journey through breast cancer diagnosis and treatment." While this book may not be the most comprehensive one you will find (as that is not its purpose), you will find it to be very "patient-friendly," containing less medical jargon and providing substantial amounts of reference for the average person to be able to comprehend.

As change is the only constant variable that time brings, what may hold true now might be susceptible to change tomorrow, given my years of practice in the field of breast cancer and my expertise in anything closely (even remotely) related to the matter, this book will surely hold some value for you. If you want the latest information and breakthroughs regarding breast cancer, then http://BreastCancerHelpCenter.org/sign-up now and see for yourself that there is indeed life after breast cancer.

I hope that by reading this book, you'll change your perspective, not just regarding your situation but your outlook on life as a whole. Breast cancer is indeed a life changing disease —but only if you allow it to be so. Armed with the proper knowledge and necessary precautions, take your fight against breast cancer aggressively and live to tell about it. For all your inquiries on breast cancer, feel free to send me an email.

All the best,
Dr. Chris Charlton
drchris@breastcancerhelpcenter.org

TABLE OF CONTENTS

CHAPTER 1 - INTRODUCTION

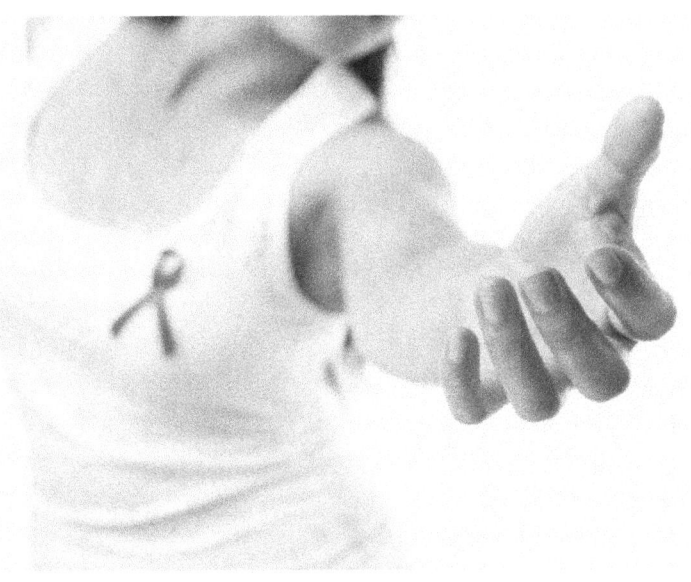

If you are reading this book, it means you or someone you love has been afflicted with this disease and you want and need to know more about it. This book is not meant to be treated as medical advice but more importantly, should be used to educate and help you and your loved ones in making the journey through breast cancer treatment and diagnosis a lot less difficult than it has to be. It should be used as a reference, which will help make visits to your doctor much more meaningful and also allow you to ask more useful questions during these trying times. This book is intended for patients with early stage breast cancer, which we define as Stage 1, 2 or 3. It will not be the most complete or comprehensive book but it is designed to help you in more simple reader-friendly terms. In the future, we will follow up with information on Stage 4 cancer because this is a very different topic with different goals.

CHAPTER 2 - BREAST CANCER BASICS AND FACTS

Breast cancer is a disease of the breast where there is an abnormal growth of breast cells. When there is uncontrolled growth, this is referred to as a malignant tumor and breast cancer is the uncontrolled growth of breast cells. Here are some basic facts to consider:

Basic Facts of Breast Cancer
» It is one of the most common malignancies in the U.S. It is expected that approximately 240,000 people will be diagnosed with breast cancer in the U.S. each year.
» We expect more than 1.3 million people will be diagnosed with breast cancer worldwide each year.
» There will also be approximately 40,000 deaths related to breast cancer in the U.S. this year.

What happens to cause breast cancer? There can be many risk factors that can increase one's likelihood of developing breast cancer; however, the actual event leading to the development of breast cancer in most patients is unknown. If the patient has a genetic mutation, which increases the risk of developing breast cancer, then we can feel fairly confident this is the likely cause. However, many times patients will ask me "Why did I get breast cancer"? I can go through various risk factors but it basically comes down to, "I do not know or bad luck". Breast cancer may have been present 3-5 years before a diagnosis was possible.

There are, however, risk factors that will increase someone's likelihood of developing breast cancer. Here are a few, as well as some facts about breast cancer:

Risk Factors of Breast Cancer
» The major risk factor in the development of breast cancer is being a woman. A woman's chances of developing breast cancer in her life are 1 in 8, which equates to a 12% lifetime risk.
» As women become older, they will also have an increased risk of developing breast cancer.
» Approximately 1% of breast cancers occur in males.
» Patients who have already had breast cancer also remain at slight increased risk of development of new breast cancers.
» A family history of breast cancer will slightly increase a person's risk of developing breast cancer. If you have a sister, mother or a daughter who has had breast cancer, then your risk of developing it is slightly greater than the general population.
» For patients who are overweight, you tend to produce more estrogen. Fat cells produce estrogen and many breast cancers are fed by estrogen. So being overweight is a risk factor for the development of breast cancer.
» Alcohol consumption will increase a woman's risk of developing breast cancer. Some studies have even suggested that one drink a day can increase someone's risk of developing breast cancer. Quality of life is also important. If a person enjoys one drink a day then that is reasonable. You must also enjoy your life and moderation in anything is the ultimate goal.
» Exercise may reduce breast cancer risk. The American Cancer Society has recommended people to engage in some type of

physical activity at least 5 days a week for 30-60 minutes.

» There may be a slight increased risk of breast cancer with smoking, but unlike lung cancer, smoking is not the predominant factor in increasing one's risk of breast cancer.

» Exposure to estrogen has always been a big risk for breast cancer. If you start menstruating at an early age and stop menstruating at a later age, you have more exposure to estrogen. This will increase your risk of breast cancer.

» A woman who has a full-term pregnancy before the age of 30 will have a lower risk of developing breast cancer. Women who never had a full-term pregnancy will have a higher risk of breast cancer.

» Patients with abnormal genetic mutations, the BRCA-1 and BRCA-2 gene have a much higher risk of breast cancer.

» There are also some cultural differences in the development of breast cancer. There's a slight increased risk of breast cancer in Caucasian women compared to African-American women. Patients of Hispanic and Asian descent do have a lower risk of breast cancer. It is interesting to note that although Caucasian and African-American receive mammograms on an equal basis, African-American patients tend to have a worse outcome because the follow-up on abnormal mammogram or the time it takes to receive treatment is delayed for African-American patients. So, the risk of dying from breast cancer tends to be higher in African-American patients.

Signs and Symptoms:

1. The big one to look for is a change in the breast.

13

2. Some patients may experience pain.
3. Some notice a lump or have a bloody nipple discharge.

There are different tests, which can be used to image the breasts. The three most common are mammograms, sonograms and MRIs. The general recommendation is that patients who are over the age of 40 should have annual clinical breast exams by a physician as well as a mammogram.

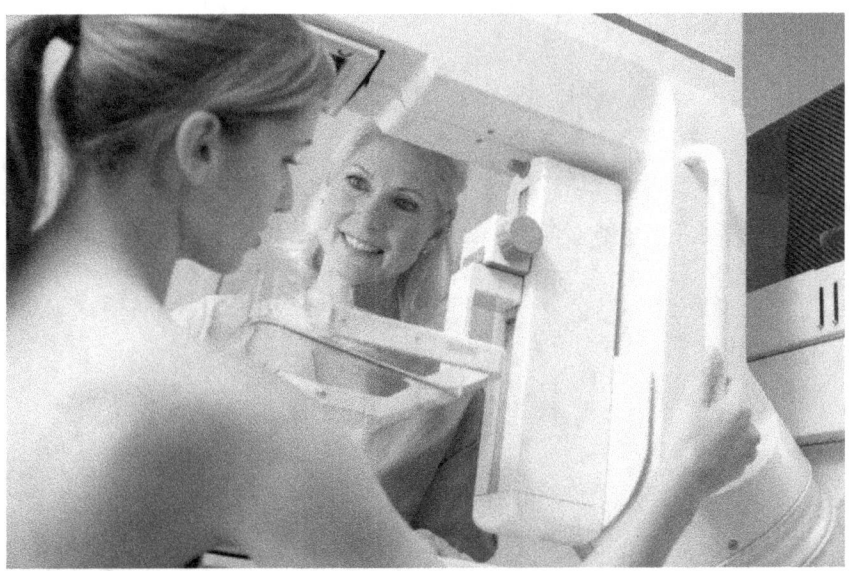

Frequently, this is a screening mammogram, which is a mammogram with two different pictures. Sometimes an abnormality is found on a screening mammogram and a diagnostic mammogram may allow the radiologist to look closer at certain suspicious areas. Again, over the age of 40 a patient should have a mammogram and physical exam every year.

Another test that could be helpful in diagnosing breast cancer is a sonogram and these are frequently used as an adjunct to a mammogram. A sonogram can be helpful in determining if a growth in the breast is fluid filled versus solid. A fluid filled growth is more likely to be a cyst whereas as a solid growth is more concerning for a malignancy. Again the sonogram is used more in conjunction with mammograms. At times I have seen a patient who has a lump, a totally normal mammogram but an abnormal sonogram.

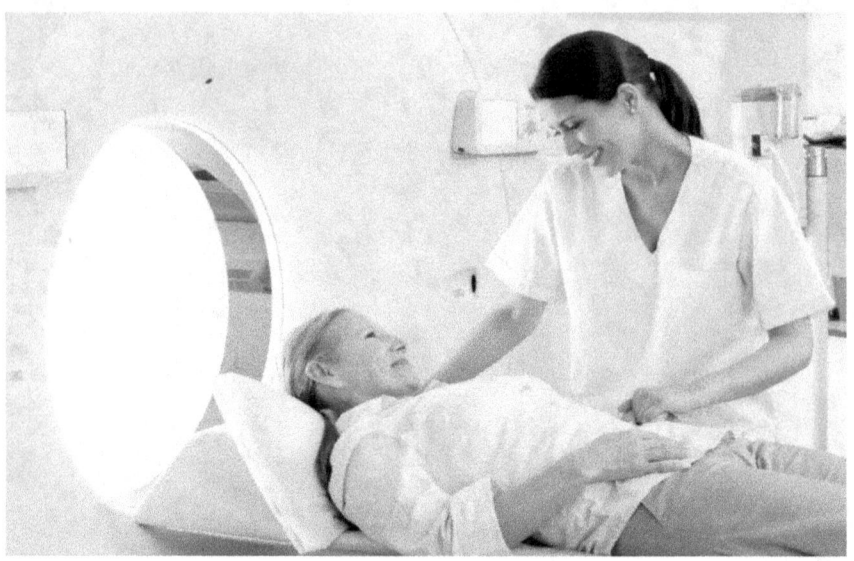

More and more physicians are starting to use MRIs in detections of breast cancers. This is a little bit controversial and you will see some physicians, breast surgeons, radiologists not placing a lot of emphasis on MRIs. MRIs can be useful in detecting abnormalities in dense breasts but they can also be used by the surgeons to see the extent of the breast cancer and give an estimate of size of the breast cancer. Some patients do not like MRIs because of the enclosed space and patients who are claustrophobic find this uncomfortable.

Once an abnormality is detected on mammogram, the findings will be labeled into one of seven categories which will guide your doctor recommendation on how to proceed. This is the **BIRADS score**:

BIRADS Score
» **Category 0**: If you're assigned this category this means the radiologist needs more information. The assessment of what is going on with your breast is incomplete so you need additional studies. They do not have the information to make a good assessment.
» **Category 1**: If you are assigned Category 1 this is negative. There is really nothing abnormal seen on the breast.
» **Category 2**: There is something going on in the breast but it is just a normal variant and likely a benign finding. The radiologist is not worried at this time. Category 1 and Category 2 are considered no evidence of malignancy.
» **Category 3**: There is something a little abnormal in the mammogram but it is likely benign and frequently at this time the radiologist will recommend a follow-up within a few months.
» **Category 4**: There is a suspicious abnormality. The radiologist is concerned and they feel that this should be addressed without waiting and a biopsy should be conducted.
» **Category 5**: There is a finding that is very suggestive of malignancy and action in the form of a biopsy+ should be taken immediately.
» **Category 6**: Occurs when a known malignancy is present already.

Once you have an abnormal finding on a mammogram, sonogram, or MRI, the important thing to do is a biopsy and frequently a biopsy is performed by a radiologist. There are two types of biopsy performed by a radiologist. One is an ultrasound guided biopsy that uses the sonogram to guide the position of the needle for the biopsy. The other biopsy technique is stereotactic biopsy. This is a little bit more of a trickier biopsy that is performed on a special table by the radiologists. This is frequently used to biopsy calcium deposits seen on a mammogram. Calcium deposits can be an indication of a malignancy in the breast but it can also be an indication of a benign findings. When a radiologist sees concerning calcium deposits on a mammogram frequently a stereotactic biopsy is performed at that time.

Sometimes the radiologist for one reason or the other is not able to obtain a good biopsy of the abnormality found. In this case an excisional biopsy is performed and this is done by a surgeon. It can be done in the office or the operating room where they make a small incision and do a bigger biopsy. This is not removing the cancer or abnormality. The main purpose is to make a diagnosis and the most convenient biopsy which achieves this goal is the best.

Once a biopsy proves breast cancer, the patient is then referred to a surgeon. If you are referred to a surgeon, here are some things to keep in mind:

Things to Keep in Mind When Referred to a Surgeon
» The surgeon should be board-certified and has done a fellowship in breast surgery, or a general surgeon who has dealt with a lot of breast cancer.

» The referral and the appointment with the surgeon does not have to be the next day. If it takes 1-2 weeks to find a surgeon in your area with whom you are comfortable, it is ok.

» The results from pathology take time. It is not as easy as looking at the results. They must be interpreted in the context of your individual case.

» It is important to remember that breast cancer, although starting in the breast, can actually be a systemic disease —a disease of the entire body.

There will also be several different health professionals involved in your care. The first is usually the radiologist who has interpreted your mammogram, sonogram and MRI if necessary and frequently performed the biopsy. The next is the surgeon who will remove the cancer from the breast and also examine the lymph nodes under the arm. A pathologist is a physician you will never meet but who is extremely important. The pathologist reviews the breast cancer providing information regarding its characteristics and also determines if there is lymph node involvement by the breast cancer. The medical oncologist is the cancer specialist who after your surgery or sometimes even before your surgery will administers chemotherapy if needed and anti-hormonal therapy if needed. The radiation oncologist is the physician who will treat the breast cancer with radiation if needed. So there may be two oncologists involved in your treatment; the medical oncologist for chemotherapy and hormonal therapy, and the radiation oncologist for radiation. Many patients will also have a plastic surgeon. Although the plastic surgeon does not directly deal with the treatment of breast cancer they certainly work with the surgeon in reconstruction for those patients who undergo removal of the breast.

Frequently performed by the surgeon or the medical oncologists is something we refer to as staging. In this book I have listed the various stages of breast cancer. There are **5 stages**: **Stage 0, 1, 2, 3** and **4**. If you cannot read the following graphic, be sure to visit us at http://BreastCancerHelpCenter.org/stages to see the full size version.

Stage 0
- Abnormal or cancer cells are present in either the lining of a breast **lobule** or a **duct,** but they have not spread to the surrounding fatty tissue.
- This stage is also called the lobular carcinoma in situ (LCIS), or ductal carcinoma in situ (DCIS).

Stage I
- Cancer has spread from the lobules or ducts to nearby tissue in the breast.
- At this stage and beyond, breast cancer is considered to be **invasive**. The **tumor** is 2 cm or less in diameter (approximately 1 inch or less); cancer has not spread to the **lymph nodes**.

Stage II
- In this stage, the tumor can range from about 2 cm to less than 5 cm in diameter (approximately 1 to 2 inches).;
- Sometimes lymph nodes may not be involved.

Stage IIIA
- In this stage, the tumor is 5 cm or greater in diameter (approximately 2 inches or greater);
- or the tumor may be of any size where cancer cells have grown extensively into axillary (underarm) lymph nodes.

Stage IIIB/C
- Known as locally advanced cancer;
- tumor may be of any size but has spread into the skin of the breast, tissues of the chest wall or lymph nodes near the collar bone.

Stage IV
- Known as **metastatic**;
- cancer has spread from the breast to other parts of the body, such as bone, liver, lung or brain.

In this book we are concerned with **stages 0 1, 2** and **3**. **Stage 4** means the cancer has moved to another part of the body.

The staging is based on the AJCC system

Evaluation of Cancer based on the following criteria	DESCRIPTION
T Category	The T component is defined by the size or contiguous extension of the primary tumor. The roles of the size component and the extent of contiguous spread in defining T are specifically defined for each cancer site.
N Category	The N component is defined by the absence, or presence and extent of cancer in the regional draining lymph nodes. Nodal involvement is categorized by the number of positive nodes and for certain cancer sites by the involvement of specific regional nodal groups.
M Category	The M component is defined by the absence or presence of distant spread or metastases, generally in locations to which the cancer spread by vascular channels, or by lymphatics beyond the nodes defined as 'regional.

Each T, N and M category is further defined by numbers that further showcase the extent of cancer	DESCRIPTION
Primary Tumor (T)	• T1, T2, T3, T4: Increasing size and/or local extension of the primary tumor

	• T0: No evidence of primary tumor • TX: Primary tumor cannot be assessed • Tis: Carcinoma in situ
Regional Lymph Nodes (N)	• N0: No regional lymph node metastases • N1, N2, N3: Increasing number or extent of regional lymph node involvement • NX: Regional lymph nodes cannot be assessed
Distant Metastasis (M)	• M0: No distant metastasis • M1: Distant metastasis present

This system assigns a stage of the cancer based on the size of the tumor, how many lymph nodes are involved, and if the cancer has moved to another parts of the body.

To fully stage a patient, it is important to make sure there is no spread of the cancer to another part of the body. Guidelines from the NCCN which is a cancer guideline authority and the American Society of Clinical Oncology (ASCO) will state that patients who have Stage 1 or even Stage 2 breast cancer may not need to undergo CAT scans, bone scans, abdominal ultrasounds, chest X-rays or PET scans because they have an early stage breast cancer and the chance that this has moved to other parts of the body is small. I tend to have a different view on this. You cannot fully determine the stage unless you have confirmed there is no spread of cancer to another part of the body. In most of my patients with an invasive breast cancer, I will do a CAT scan of the chest and abdomen and a bone scan which are the preferred choices. This looks at the lung, liver and bone –the three favorite places for breast cancer to spread. A PET scan is another option which also looks at the whole body.

If there is no convincing evidence of cancer, then I feel comfortable saying, "This is an early stage breast cancer". Several patients throughout my career who were presumed to have early stage breast cancer were found to have spread of the cancer to another part of the body. I feel it is important to know this upfront because it offers prognostic information to the patient and also allows us to intervene in a more appropriate manner. Again, I differ at times from than the national guidelines but unless you fully know there is no concrete evidence of spread of the cancer then you cannot accurately determine the stage.

I have discussed some of the imaging studies that can be used such as CAT scans or bone scans and this is the preferred method. PET scans have become popular and many patients will request a PET scan. I always inform patients that there can be false negatives because PET scans may not pick up abnormalities less than 5mm in size. Nevertheless, a PET scan does remain an option. Sometimes insurance companies especially in this new age of medicine will not approve of CAT scans, bone scans, or PETS. In that case, I will frequently do a chest x-ray or abdominal ultrasound which is not preferable but sometimes the only option we have. The AJCC mentioned earlier with regards to staging stands for the American Joint Committee on Cancer and they are the ones who came up with the T-tumor, N-node, M-metastasis (TNM). At the end of the book there will be a copy of the AJCC staging system. Remember, this can only be accurately determined after surgery and CAT scans, bone scans, or PET scans are complete.

CHAPTER 3 - TYPES OF BREAST CANCER

DCIS: This is stage 0 breast cancer and where we want to detect breast cancer. The reason we do mammograms and sonograms is to find breast cancer when it is in situ. In situ means the cancer is sitting on the surface of the breast duct and has not invaded into the breast tissue which increases the risk of spread. It is not an invasive cancer. It is treated and normally cured with surgery alone plus or minus radiation. Anyone who is diagnosed with DCIS (Duct Cell Carcinoma In Situ) will not require chemotherapy. If a patient has DCIS and is left untreated, it will eventually become an invasive cancer. The risk of DCIS spreading to another part of the body such as the lung, liver or bones is 1%. If properly treated with surgery and radiation the risk of it returning in the breast, in my experience, is less than 10%.

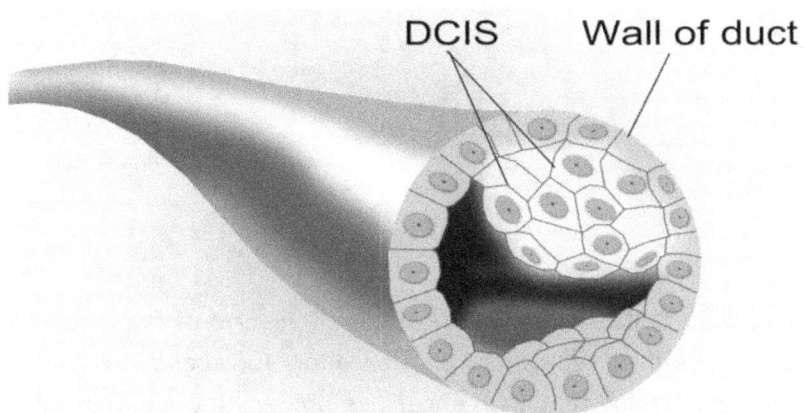

LCIS: Another variant of breast cancer is referred to as LCIS or Lobular Carcinoma In Situ. This is also called lobular neoplasia. Again this is not a breast cancer but abnormal growth on the lobules of the breast. Sometimes it is really helpful to look at a picture of the breast. The breast is divided into lobules, the milk-producing glands of the breast, when the milk is expressed from the breast it drains from lobules towards ducts and the ducts converge to the nipple. Patients who are diagnosed with this do have an increased risk of developing breast cancer although lobular neoplasia is not breast cancer in itself. No surgery is needed for this condition but careful observation is needed.

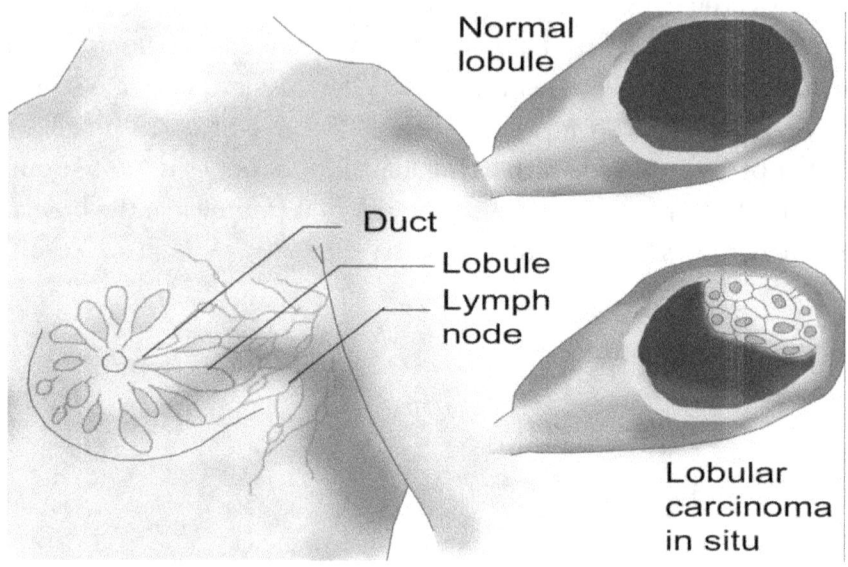

Normal lobule

Duct

Lobule

Lymph node

Lobular carcinoma in situ

Invasive Duct Cell Cancer: The most common form of breast cancer we see is invasive duct cell cancer. This accounts for about 75% of invasive cancers. This means that the cancer has broken through a specific milk duct into the surrounding breast tissue where it can be exposed to blood vessels and lymphatics and potentially move to another part of the body. There are variants of invasive breast cancer which we will discuss and these are determined by the pathologist examining the breast tissue. Some patients may have a combination of the variants.

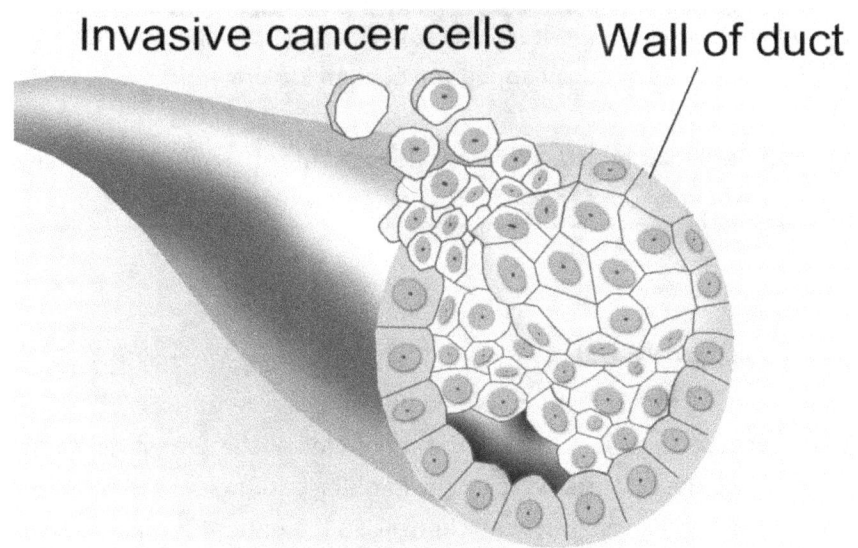

Invasive cancer cells   **Wall of duct**

Variants of Invasive Breast Cancer
» **Cribriform carcinoma**: This looks like nests of cells which invade between the tissues and have holes between the tumor cells. An invasive cancer, which has an acribriform component, tends to represent a better prognostic variant.
» **Tubular carcinoma**: This is a very favorable form of breast cancer where the tumor cells form tubules. How do we know this is the case? The pathologist tells us. Oncologists love to see tubular cancers because overall they do a lot better. It's still an invasive cancer but a better variant.
» **Mucinous carcinoma** or **colloid carcinoma**: This tends to be a less aggressive more favorable variant of cancer where the tumor cells are surrounded by a mucous substance called mucin. Some cancers may be pure mucinous cancers or just have part of the cancer that has the mucinous feature. Again this is a better acting breast cancer.
» **Medullary cancers** or **medullary carcinoma**: This is rare and

again, tends to be less aggressive rarely moving outside the breast. It has a mushy appearance when looking at it.

» **Papillary carcinoma**: This is the variant of invasive duct cell carcinoma which tends to affect older women.

Invasive lobular carcinoma: This accounts for about 15% of invasive cancers and is the second most common invasive cancer. It is called lobular because the cancer starts in the lobules of the breast which again drain into the ducts. It tends to occur in older patients and is treated the same way as an invasive duct cell cancer. So if a patient is diagnosed with invasive duct cell or lobular cancer they are treated the same for the most part. The variants I spoke of previously are generally associated with invasive duct cell carcinomas.

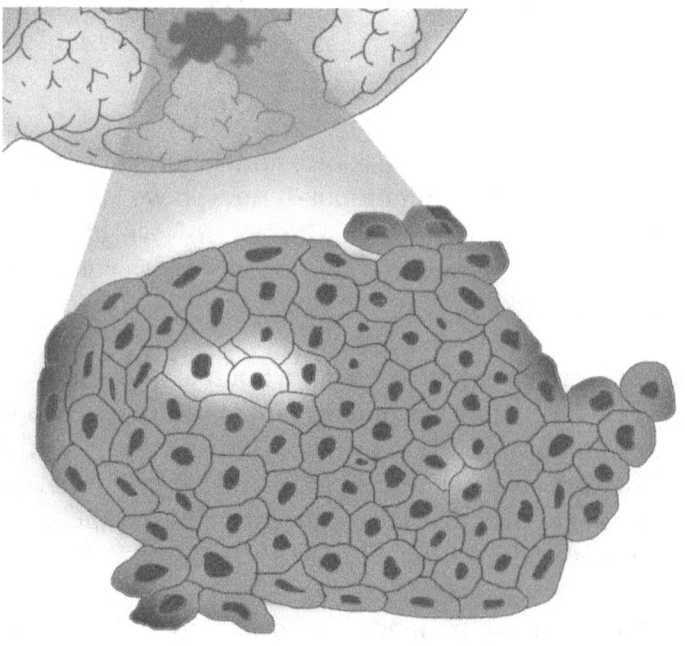

Triple Negative Breast Cancer: Another form of invasive breast cancer I want to mention is referred to as triple negative breast cancer. We have learned more about this over the past few years. This is a very aggressive form of breast cancer that does not express estrogen or progesterone receptors and is also HER2 negative. Please understand that when someone is diagnosed with a triple negative breast cancer they will frequently require chemotherapy. It is also a breast cancer which does not respond to hormonal therapy which we will also discuss later in the book.

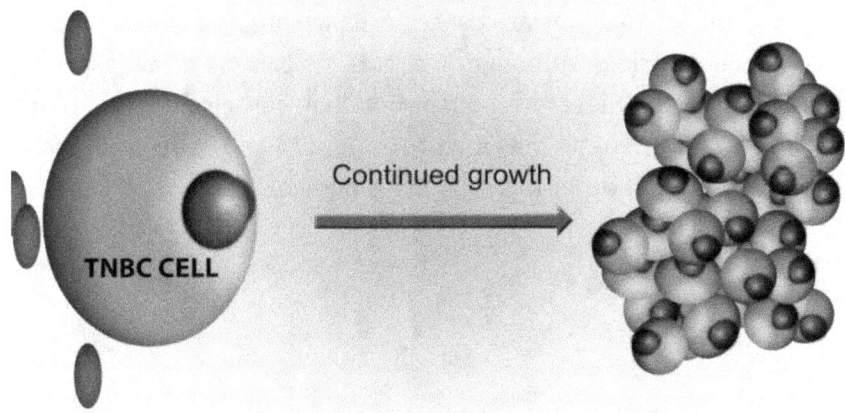

Inflammatory Breast Cancer: This is an unusual but very aggressive form of breast cancer. This cancer presents with changes to the skin of the breast where the breast can frequently become red and also have an orange peel feel and look. It is referred to as peau d'orange, which is French for orange peel. This occurs because the tumor has invaded into the lymphatic system of the skin.

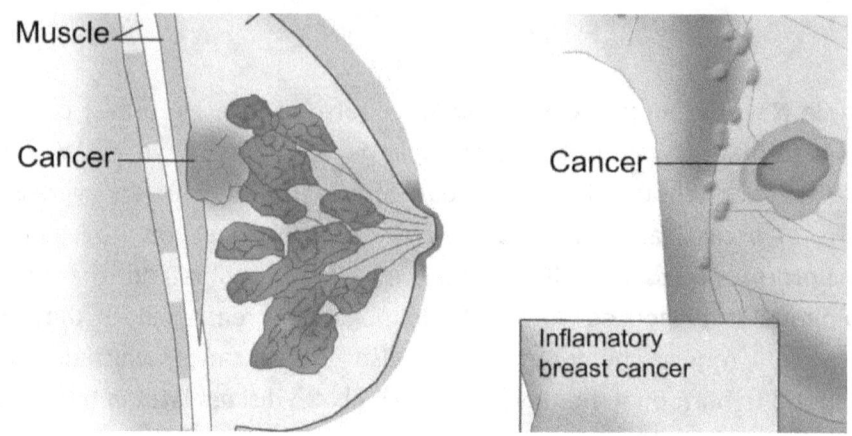

Muscle

Cancer

Cancer

Inflamatory breast cancer

Phyllodes Tumor: This is a rare cancer usually confined to the breast and rarely moves outside. Although we classify this as a breast cancer, frequently many of these are benign but they can also be malignant or even part benign part malignant. Generally, no chemotherapy or additional treatment other than surgery is needed for these cancers.

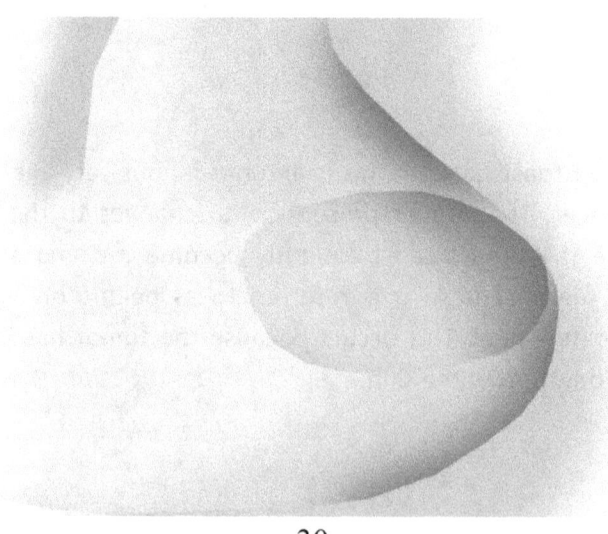

Male Breast Cancers: As stated before 1% of breast cancers in the U.S. affect men. Men have small amounts of breast tissue so there is obviously less risk but some risk factors which do increase the chances of men developing breast cancer are gynecomastia which is basically the technical term for enlarged breasts. This can occur with certain genetic mutations, and also obesity. Breast cancer is treated the same way in both men and women.

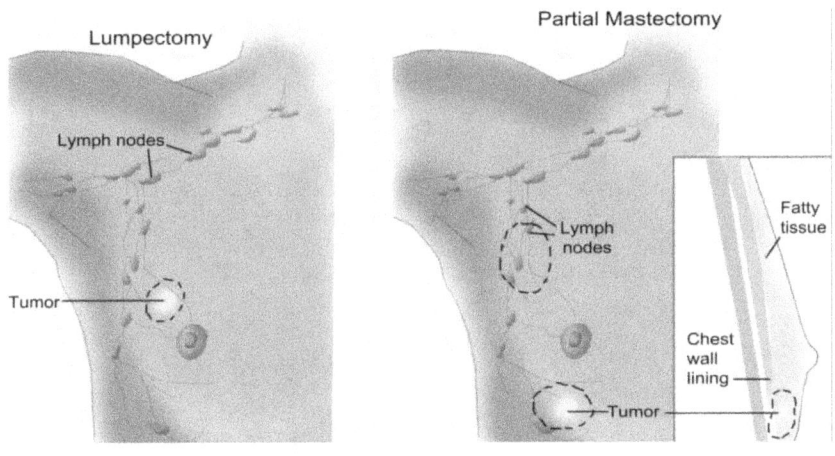

Angiosarcoma: This is an invasive breast carcinoma in patients with prior exposure to chest wall or breast radiation in their life.

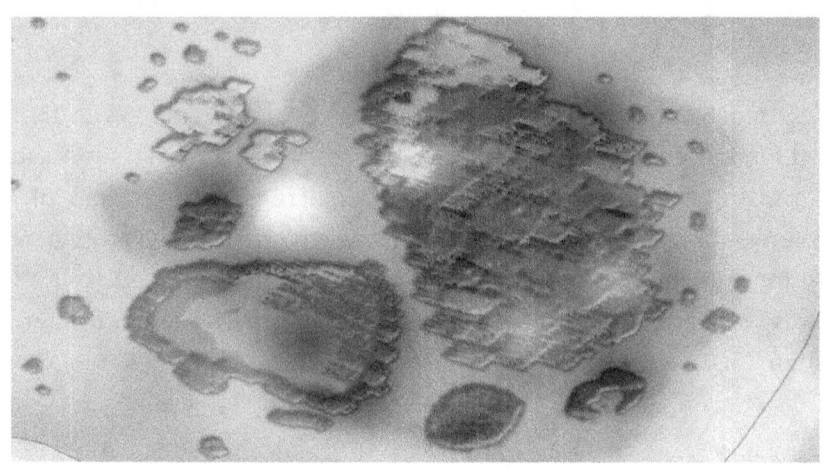

Chapter 4 – Surgery

The goal of surgery is complete removal of the breast cancer. The type of surgery that you have does not influence if you will need chemotherapy or anti-hormonal therapy down the line. The reason for this is that breast cancer is a disease of the body not just the breasts. The surgery is designed to treat the breast not the rest of the body. Breast tissue drains to lymph nodes under the arm so when you have a breast cancer on your left breast it will most likely drain to the lymph nodes under the left arm. Mammogram, sonogram or MRIs do not give the precise measurement of the tumor. Only surgery will tell you the exact size of the tumor.

The surgeon will also assess the lymph nodes. This is important for two reasons: prognostic information and removal of any cancer. Prognostic information is important because the more lymph node involvement with cancer the worse the prognosis is. By assessing the lymph nodes we have prognostic information but the surgeon has also performed a therapeutic procedure by removing the next logical place the cancer would go.

There are three main types of surgery

Biopsy: We have previously discussed the excisional biopsy which may be done if the radiologist is unable to do a stereotactic or ultrasound-guided biopsy during the diagnosis phase. The excisional biopsy is not designed to remove the tumor and the lymph nodes.

Lumpectomy: sometimes referred to as a partial mastectomy is the preferred method of breast cancer surgery these days. This removes the cancer lump without removing the entire breast. This is possible if the cancer can be removed with surrounding normal breast tissue. There should be a space —referred to as a margin of at least 3 mm between the breast tissues and where the cancer was removed. This gives us confidence that all the cancer was removed and no cells were left. By removing a little bit of extra normal tissue the surgeon will feel more secure they have removed all of the cells.

Mastectomy: There are two types of mastectomy performed today. One is the modified radical mastectomy and the other is skin-sparing mastectomy. The radical mastectomy was used in the past and that is where the breast and the underlying pectoralis muscle, which is the muscle under the breast, were removed. This is no longer done as it was extremely deforming to a patient. The decision whether to proceed with a mastectomy is frequently made on the size of the cancer, location, and the patient's preference. If the cancer is too big, a lumpectomy with clear margins may not be feasible then a mastectomy must be performed. The surgeon should tell the patient if they do not feel there is a good likelihood they can perform a lumpectomy and still leave the patient with a good cosmetic outcome.

Basic Facts on Mastectomy
» One disadvantage of a mastectomy is there is usually a 2-3 days stay in the hospital and patients may have small drains which are connected under the skin to drain fluid which can build up after

surgery. These usually will remain for about 1 - 2 weeks and can be very uncomfortable.

» Now, some patients who undergo a mastectomy will also sometimes elect to have the other breast removed as a precaution. The other breast may not be involved with cancer but patients want it as prevention. Remember if you have cancer in one breast you also have a slightly increased risk of developing a new cancer on the other breast. The procedure where both breasts are removed is called a bilateral mastectomy. This is a personal decision but I must admit, I see it more often these days. Patients have told me that going through the stress of cancer on one side, they do not want a "déjà vu" on the other side.

» Also something that is commonly misunderstood is that cancer on one breast rarely moves to the other breast. If cancer develops on the other breast, it is most likely a new breast cancer unrelated to the original cancer.

» Reconstruction following mastectomy is a very personal decision and has no bearing on the cancer. It is important to find a plastic surgeon that you are comfortable with as this can be a long process. The plastic surgeon will frequently keep pictures of their work which you can view. Sometimes reconstruction can be performed or at least started at the time of surgery where an implant can be placed under the pectoralis muscle which is the muscle behind the breast or they can place what we refer to as a tissue expander which is basically an expander which can be filled with fluid to stretch the skin. After several months, the expander can be removed and the final implant placed.

Lymph Node Assessment: As part of the surgery, a lymph node assessment will be performed. Sometimes this is done before the surgery and sometimes after the surgery.

Lymph nodes are small glands throughout the body that are connected to the lymphatic system, which is similar to the blood system. The lymphatic system does drain into the blood or the circulatory system. The most common way to assess the lymph nodes, which lie under the arm, is using a procedure called sentinel lymph node sampling. To put this simply, it is a method to remove the most likely lymph node or lymph nodes the breast cancer would spread to. Previously all of the lymph nodes under the arm were removed but we know this increases the risk of arm swelling —lymphedema— and also puts the patient through extensive surgery.

The sentinel lymph node procedure allows the surgeon to remove the lymph node where the cancer is most likely to travel. The procedure is performed by the radiologist or surgeon who will inject the tumor of the breast with a radioactive dye and this travels presumably where the cancer would travel to the lymph nodes under the arm. The lymph node, which contains the most dye and which is most radioactive, is removed.

Some surgeons will perform the sentinel lymph node procedure at the same time as the breast surgery and others prefer to do it before the breast surgery. Doing this before the breast cancer surgery allows the surgeon to be prepared to take additional lymph nodes (an auxiliary dissection) at the time of the final surgery if there is cancer involved with the sentinel lymph node. However the downside to doing this is that there are two surgical procedures, which mean two general anesthetics. Again the goal of sentinel lymph node is to allow fewer nodes to be taken. It is not a perfect procedure and sometimes fails. This means there is a small possibility lymph nodes could contain cancer which were not the sentinel lymph node. It could be missed. This is unusual but it is possible. However during the surgery, the surgeon will do a thorough exam and any suspicious findings such as abnormal lymph nodes will be removed.

If the breast cancer surgery and lymph node sampling are performed at the same time, a procedure called a frozen section is performed by the pathologist. This is where the pathologist will look at the margins of the lumpectomy specimen and the sentinel lymph node while the patient is asleep in surgery. If they see that the margins at lumpectomy are involved they will tell the surgeon who will remove additional tissue at that time. If the sentinel lymph node seems to be involved with cancer then the surgeon will remove additional lymph nodes and make sure that all of the cancer is removed and no additional lymph nodes are involved. Frozen section sampling is extremely helpful as it can prevent a person from additional surgery but it is by no means perfect. Frozen section is a technique that allows basically a very cursory look at the specimen.

It takes several days for the specimens from surgery to be prepared for the pathologists to examine. When looking at the specimens they may see there is an involved margin with the cancer and the patient would have to return for additional surgery. They may also discover the sentinel lymph node thought to have no cancer during frozen section actually has cancer. This may also require another surgery to remove additional lymph nodes as a precaution to make sure all of the disease is removed. If the sentinel lymph node is not involved with cancer it is unlikely that any additional lymph nodes will need to be removed.

CHAPTER 5 - UNDERSTANDING THE PATHOLOGY REPORT – WHAT IS REALLY IMPORTANT

The pathology report is the most important piece of information your oncologist and surgeon will need. It gives information about your cancer that will be used to determine the next step in your treatment. Pathology reports are in many ways very confusing however the College of American Pathologists (CAP) have set guidelines which standardize pathology reports from one place to the next. Meaning, the pathology report from one hospital should give you the same information as the pathology reports from another.

Be sure to request your pathology report so you can ask educated questions of your doctor and discuss your course of treatment. The following example and explanation is no substitute for talking with your physician – it's meant to supplement your discussion and give you a frame of reference to understand the next step in your course of treatment.

A pathology report is a description of cells and tissues made by a pathologist based on microscopic evidence – it's a long list of technical terms and measurements. Below is an example but if you cannot see it very well, be sure to take a look online:
http://BreastCancerHelpCenter.org/pathology

SUMMARY OF PATHOLOGIC FEATURES: BREAST CARCINOMA

Pathologic Stage: -pT1c, pN0 (i-)(sn)
Based on AJCC TNM Staging Manual, 7th ed.
Procedure: -Partial Mastectomy with wire guided localization.
Lymph Node Sampling: -Sentinel lymph nodes.
Specimen laterality: -Left.
Tumor Location: -6:00 o' clock, 6 centimeters from nipple.

TUMOR CHARACTERISTICS:
Tumor Size (Invasive component): -1.8 centimeters in greatest dimension.
Tumor Focality: -Single focus of invasive carcinoma.

HISTOPATHOLOGIC FEATURES
Histologic Type: -Invasive ductal carcinoma (no special type).

Combined Histologic Grade (Nottingham Grade): -Grade 3 (high grade).

Tubule formation: -Score 3 (Breakpoints: >75% = score 1; 10-75% = score 2; <10% = score 3).

Nuclear grade: -Score 3 (Three tiers based on degree of pleomorphism grade 1 showing little nuclear variation and grade 3 showing marked variation).

Mitotic Rate: -Score 3; 39 mitoses per 10 HPF (Breakpoints, based on 0.54 mm field diameter: 0-8 mitoses = score 1; 9-16 mitoses = score 2; >26 mitoses = score 3).

Peripheral tumor margins: -Circumscribed
Lymphovascular Invasion: -Not Identified
Venous (Large Vessel) Invasion: -Not Identified
Lymphatic (Small Vessel) Invasion: -Not Identified
Perineural Invasion: -Not Identified
Ductal Carcinoma In Situ: -Present, solid type(s), high nuclear grade, without an extensive intraductal component.
Necrosis: -Present, involving invasive carcinoma (2% of invasive tumor).
Surgical Margins: -Uninvolved by invasive and in-situ carcinoma; for invasive carcinoma, anterior margin uninvolved by 0.2 centimeter; for DCIS, Posterior margin uninvolved by 0.1 cm.

	INVASIVE CARCINOMA	DCIS
Anterior:	Free by 0.2 cm.	Free by 0.5 cm.
Posterior:	Free by 0.6 cm.	Free by 0.1 cm.
Lateral:	Free by greater than 1.0 cm.	Free by greater than 1.0 cm.
Medial:	Free by greater than 1.0 cm.	Free by greater than 1.0 cm.
Superior:	Free by 1.1 cm.	Free by greater than 1.0 cm.
Inferior:	Free by 1.6 cm.	Free by greater than 1.0 cm.

Calcification: -Present, associated with nonneoplastic breast tissue.
Skin: -Skin is not present.
Nipple: -Nipple not present.
Skeletal Muscle: -No skeletal muscle present.
Additional Findings: -Nonproliferative fibrocystic changes, Intraductal papilloma.

REGIONAL LYMPH NODES
Number Recovered: -Two sentinel lymph node(s).
Total Number Involved: -Zero (0/2).
Other Changes in Nodes: -Reactive sinus histiocytosis, partial fatty replacement.

PREDICTIVE/PROGNOSTIC MARKERS
Specimen Studied: -Paraffin embedded tissue, Block B4.
Fixation/Duration: -10% neutral buffered formalin fixation for 26.5 hours.
Preparation adequacy: -Lesional tissue affirmatively identified on slides examined; internal controls appropriate.
Estrogen Receptor (immunostain): -POSITIVE (1+ staining in 10% of nuclei).
Progesterone Receptor (immunostain): -POSITIVE (1+ staining in 1% of nuclei).
Ki-67 proliferative rate (immunostain): -HIGH (50% of invasive tumor nuclei express Ki-67).
HER2 (ERBB2, immunostain): -EQUIVOCAL for overexpression (2+).
External controls: -High protein, intermediate protein, negative protein expression controls all satisfactory.
Internal Controls: -Native breast ducts faintly staining.
Exclusion criteria (ASCO/CAP): -None.
Staining pattern: -Circumferential but non-uniform and weak.
Staining Uniformity: -Non-uniform.
Percentage of cells staining as above: -30%
HER2 (FISH): -AMPLIFIED.

40

Let's examine the pathology report more closely. What's important on the report? What's your next step?

The report will first tell you what **type of breast cancer** *(see Histologic Type)*.

SUMMARY OF PATHOLOGIC FEATURES: BREAST CARCINOMA	
Histologic Type	Invasive ductal carcinoma (no special type).

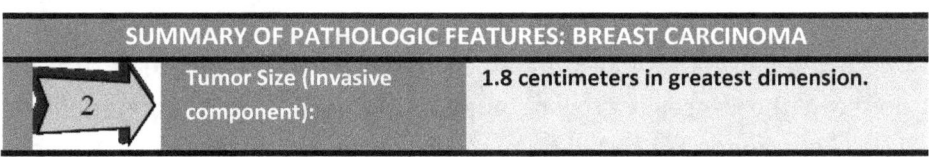

You may already know this from the biopsy but again, this will confirm whether it is a duct cell cancer, lobular cancer, tubular or even1 in situ cancer —DCIS. It will also give you the definitive size. Again, there may be many sizes on the path report such as the size of the lump that is removed but the only size that is really important is the **size of the invasive component** *(see Tumor Size)*.

SUMMARY OF PATHOLOGIC FEATURES: BREAST CARCINOMA	
Tumor Size (Invasive component):	1.8 centimeters in greatest dimension.

We do not really care about the size of the in situ component whether it is 1 cm or 10 cm makes no difference. However, we do need to know the size of the invasive component. The next factor to look at is the **grade of the tumor** *(see Combined Histologic Grade)*.

41

SUMMARY OF PATHOLOGIC FEATURES: BREAST CARCINOMA		
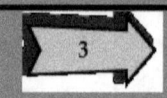	Combined Histologic Grade (Nottingham Grade):	Grade 3 (high grade).

Frequently, patients get confused between grade and stage. These are totally different things.

Grade is how aggressive the cancer is, where **Stage** *(see* Pathologic Stage*)* is how advanced the cancer is.

SUMMARY OF PATHOLOGIC FEATURES: BREAST CARCINOMA		
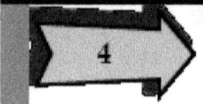	Pathologic Stage:	**pT1c, pN0 (i-)(sn)** *Based on AJCC TNM Staging Manual, 7th ed.*

The pathologist determines the grade based on different criteria such as how fast the cancer is growing and whether the cancer forms tubules. This is not important but it is important to know if your cancer is grade one, which generally means it is less aggressive, grade 2 is medium aggressiveness and grade three is a more aggressive cancer. The grade is one of the criteria used by the medical oncologist when recommending treatment. The next important section is the **margins of the tumor** *(see* Surgical Margins*)*.

	Surgical Margins:	Uninvolved by invasive and in-situ carcinoma; for invasive carcinoma, anterior margin uninvolved by 0.2 centimeter; for DCIS, Posterior margin uninvolved by 0.1 cm.
5		

I spent time discussing this in the surgery section but it is important to know that all of the cancer was microscopically removed. We want at least a 3 mm. Other physicians would say 1mm, I would use 3mm but preferably 5 mm margins. Again, a margin is the gap between all the sides of the tumor and normal breast tissue. Pathologists will give the distance in mm or cm. If the margins are not clear, they will say the margin is involved or they may say the cancer is approaching the margin or maybe less than one millimeter. This will mean additional surgery to ensure all the cancer has been removed and, in some cases, may mean a mastectomy. If for some reason the margins are closely involved but additional surgery cannot be performed then radiation may be needed as there is always a chance spare cells may have been left. The one margin that is tough to deal with is the back or the posterior margin because it backs up to the muscle of the chest wall called the pectoralis muscle. The surgeon will remove as much of the cancer as possible without removing the muscle but if the cancer is at the pectoralis muscle you may need radiation.

The **lymph node status** *(see* Regional Lymph Nodes*)* is very important.

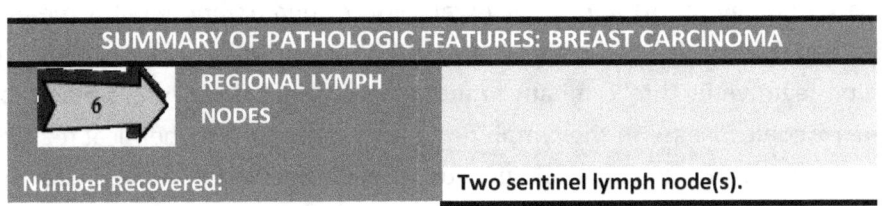

	REGIONAL LYMPH NODES	
6		
Number Recovered:		Two sentinel lymph node(s).

Total Number Involved:	Zero (0/2).
Other Changes in Nodes:	Reactive sinus histiocytosis, partial fatty replacement.

It also contributes to determining the stage of the breast cancer. On the lymph node section of the pathology report the total of nodes removed will be listed as well as the total number of nodes involved with cancer. How the cancer is involved with lymph nodes is divided into three ways: macroscopic, microscopic, and Immunohistochemical positive —I (+). This is confusing and we will go over it in detail. It should also be remembered the number of lymph nodes removed will be different among patients. Patients who only have a sentinel lymph node removed may only have one or two lymph nodes examined. However patients who have cancer involving the sentinel lymph node will have additional lymph nodes removed either at the time of surgery or with an additional surgery. The surgeon does not always know how many lymph nodes they are removing as the lymph nodes can be close to the breast tissue and may be removed as part of the breast tissue. Patients tell me, "They only removed one lymph node". Well, the pathology report says they removed 6 lymph nodes. Again, the pathology report is the bible and the final proof. Let's look at the sizes of the cancer in the lymph nodes. If there is macroscopic involvement of cancer in the lymph nodes that means the cancer in the lymph nodes is greater than 0.2 cm. Microscopic means the cancer can only be seen by the microscope and is less than 0.2 cm.

The next part is confusing and I hesitate to discuss it but you will see it in the pathology report and I really want you to understand what it means. So read this carefully. The lymph nodes if negative will be read as negative i+ or negative i-. The "i" means Immunohistochemical. If there is macro or microscopic disease in the lymph node, the Immunohistochemical feature is not used. However pathologists on all negative lymph nodes meaning

44

they cannot see any cancer even within the microscope will put a special chemical on the lymph nodes which will highlight any single or clusters of cells in the lymph node.

This is the **Immunohistochemical stain** *(see* Immunohistochemical Stain*)*.

SUMMARY OF PATHOLOGIC FEATURES: BREAST CARCINOMA	
Ki-67 proliferative rate (immunostain):	HIGH (50% of invasive tumor nuclei express Ki-67).

The problem is we do not know what those highlighted cells mean. They could be small cancer cells that have moved from the breast to the lymph node or just normal cells that have just moved from the breast to the lymph nodes from manipulation of the breast during biopsy or surgery. However, even if highlighted cells are found, the lymph node is still considered a negative or not involved lymph node in the staging system. It will be classified as N0 (i + or -). Most oncologists look at this information but do not put a great deal of emphasis of this stain. So the question may arise—why is it even checked? Well that is a good question and no one really has an answer. Any person who can tell you exactly what these cells mean - run, they have no clue what they are talking about!   In the reference pathology report shown, the **"i" status** *(see* I Status*)* is shown with the stage.

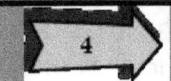

SUMMARY OF PATHOLOGIC FEATURES: BREAST CARCINOMA	
Pathologic Stage:	**pT1c, pN0 (i-)(sn)** *Based on AJCC TNM Staging Manual, 7th ed.*

Another finding you will also see within the lymph node section of the pathology report is something referred to as extra capsular extension. This means the cancer has broken through the lymph nodes. This is certainly removed by the surgeon at the time of surgery but is also another risk factor we take into consideration when deciding treatment —namely radiation in this instance.

The next important section of the pathology report is what we refer to as the **receptor status** (*see* Receptor Status).

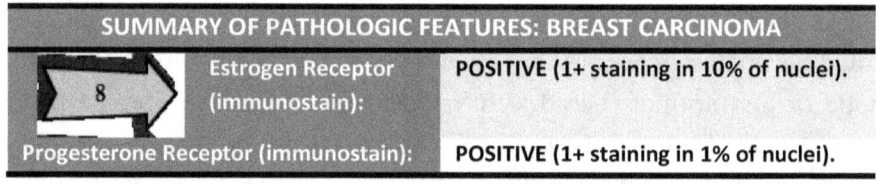

SUMMARY OF PATHOLOGIC FEATURES: BREAST CARCINOMA	
Estrogen Receptor (immunostain):	POSITIVE (1+ staining in 10% of nuclei).
Progesterone Receptor (immunostain):	POSITIVE (1+ staining in 1% of nuclei).

3Cancer cells may have receptors or almost like little baseball cups of the cell's surface. These are referred to as estrogen and progesterone receptors. When they are present it is referred to as positive. That means the breast cancer cells are fed by the female hormones estrogen and progesterone. This is a good thing. We want this. It is good for two reasons. Breast cancer cells which are fed by estrogen and progesterone tend to be less aggressive and also make a patient a candidate for the anti-hormonal pills. These pills commonly referred to as hormonal therapy and include names such as tamoxifen, Arimidex, or Femara. So it is not only a better acting breast cancer but it also gives the oncologist another option for treatment, meaning systemic treatment, because these pills go throughout the whole body. Cancer cells which do not have these hormone receptors meaning "negative" tend to be much more aggressive and do not respond to any of the pills.

The last major part of the pathology report will also be reported near the hormone receptor section of the report.

This is called **HER2NEU** or **HER2 status** *(see HER2 Status)*.

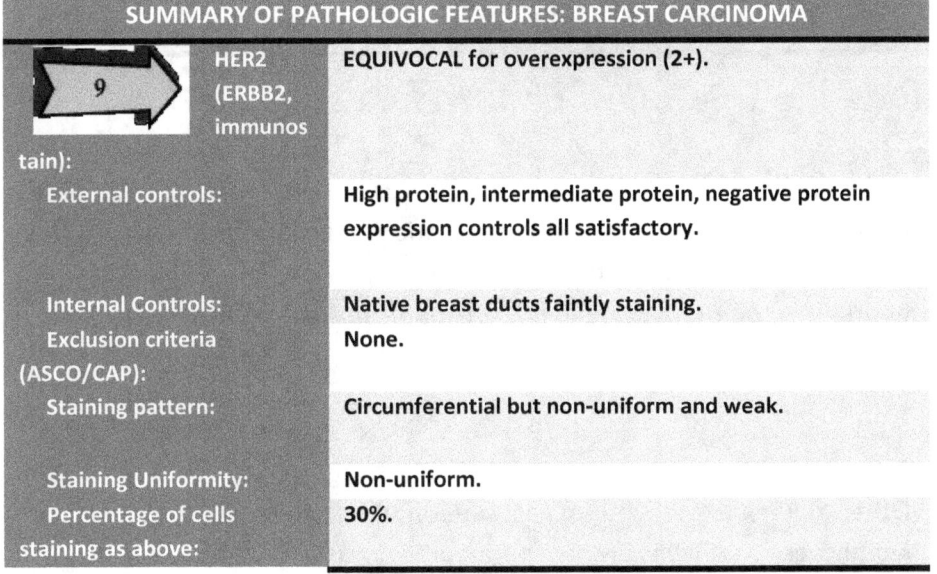

SUMMARY OF PATHOLOGIC FEATURES: BREAST CARCINOMA	
HER2 (ERBB2, immunostain):	EQUIVOCAL for overexpression (2+).
External controls:	High protein, intermediate protein, negative protein expression controls all satisfactory.
Internal Controls:	Native breast ducts faintly staining.
Exclusion criteria (ASCO/CAP):	None.
Staining pattern:	Circumferential but non-uniform and weak.
Staining Uniformity:	Non-uniform.
Percentage of cells staining as above:	30%.

This stands for human epidermal receptor 2. I am just going to refer to this as HER2. HER2 is a protein on about 20% of the breast cancer cells and makes the cancer more aggressive. On the pathology report HER2 will be reported by how intensely it stains on the cancer cells. A pathologist can put stains on the cancer cells and determine how intense they are. If they report the stain as 0 or 1+, this is negative or no HER2. If the HER2 stain is reported as 3+ then it is considered positive or yes for HER2. If the stain is 2+ it is considered indeterminate. In these cases a special test called a FISH will be performed to determine if this cancer really is HER2 positive or HER2 negative.

And the **HER2 FISH test** *(see HER2 Fish Test)* will be reported as AMPLIFIED which means HER2 positive or NOT AMPLIFIED which is HER2 negative.

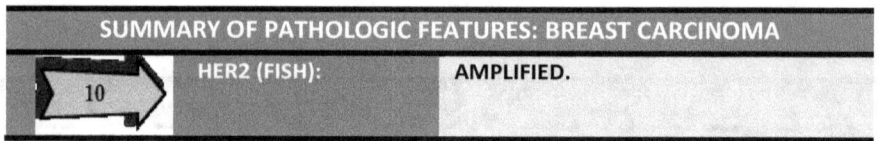

SUMMARY OF PATHOLOGIC FEATURES: BREAST CARCINOMA	
HER2 (FISH):	AMPLIFIED.

It is very important to know the HER2 status of the cancer. As you will see later it has important treatment implications. Cancers which over-express HER2 must be treated with a drug called trastuzumab or Herceptin which neutralizes the HER2 protein. It is an important part of any chemotherapy treatment.

Other findings that you might see on the pathology report include lymphovascular invasion or perineural invasion. Perineural invasion indicates there may be potential invasion around the nerves within the breast. **Lymphovascular invasion** *(see Lymphovascular Invasion)* suggest the cancer has invaded into the lymphatics (even if it has not reached the lymph nodes) or the blood vessels.

SUMMARY OF PATHOLOGIC FEATURES: BREAST CARCINOMA	
Lymphovascular invasion:	Not Identified
Venous (Large Vessel) Invasion:	Not Identified
Lymphatic (Small Vessel) Invasion:	Not Identified

These both are risk factors the oncologists will look at and take into consideration when recommending treatment. Once the information is available from the pathology report it is combined with the various x-rays that we discussed before (CAT scans, bone scans or PET scans) to determine the precise stage. Again, the **staging** is listed at the **end of the book**.

Chapter 6 - Chemotherapy

Unfortunately we must discuss the most unpopular part of this book but nevertheless an important aspect. As I have mentioned several times in this book, breast cancer is a systemic or full body disease potentially affecting the entire body not just the breast. It is very important that you think of breast cancer this way otherwise you will not understand the treatments for breast cancer. There is always the potential that breast cancer cells can escape from the breast and enter the circulatory system and then deposit in one of the solid organs. This risk is higher with lymph node involvement by cancer but it can still happen without lymph node involvement. Chemotherapy regimens are drugs which are designed to travel throughout the body and lower the risk of breast cancer cells settling in other organs.

Even with normal x-rays, CAT scans, PET scans, it does not mean there are no circulating cancer cells in the body. These cells are too small to detect with today's technology. When we can see cancer cell deposits (via x-rays, etc.) in another part of the body it is too late for cure. This is already stage 4. The purpose of chemotherapy is to decrease the risk of development of stage 4 disease by killing these microscopic cells. How do we know these microscopic cells are floating in the body? We don't! By looking at your pathology report and perhaps performing other tests, the medical oncologist will make an assessment to the risk of these cells being in the body. But regardless, we can never be sure.

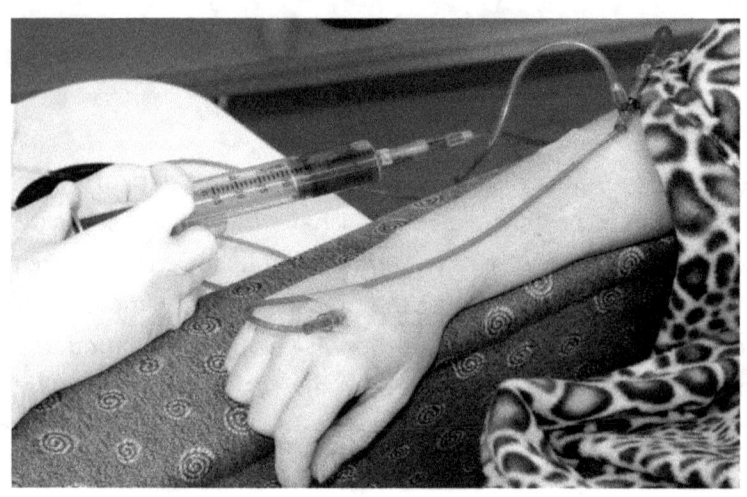

The purpose of chemotherapy and hormonal therapy is to decrease your risk of future disease. It should be considered as a form of insurance. In some patients who are considered low risk, there may be no need for chemotherapy. Patients have sometimes said to me "I do not want to go to chemotherapy unless the cancer comes back". This is an incorrect and a potentially deadly thought process. If cancer comes back it is more likely to be somewhere else in the body, not the breast. Let me repeat this, somewhere else in the body, not the breast. This is then a stage 4 disease and it is then too late to cure the cancer. We have one chance to be aggressive with the cancer and that is upfront not later. I have been repetitive about this as it is a very important concept to understand. Please understand this section and if you do not read it again.

There are two ways to deliver chemotherapy. The most common is referred to as **adjuvant** treatment and this is to deliver chemotherapy after the surgery has been performed. Another way to deliver chemotherapy is before surgery in order to shrink the cancer —this is called **neoadjuvant**. Indications for neoadjuvant chemotherapy are inflammatory breast cancers, large breast cancers greater than 5 cm or evidence of involved lymph nodes with cancer.

If lymph nodes are involved with breast cancer this tells us there is an increased risk that cancerous cells may have escaped towards the rest of the body. So in these situations we know that the treatment which protects the body by killing cancerous cells is chemotherapy. Upfront chemotherapy not only kills potential cells that may have escaped but also shrinks the cancer in the breast and may make it easier to operate. The biggest risk to someone with breast cancer is the movement of cancer cells to another part of the body. Occasionally, cancers which are very large (greater than 5 cm) will need to be shrunk in order for successful surgery. This may also make lumpectomy more feasible. Inflammatory breast cancer is also an indication for neoadjuvant breast cancer. Receiving chemotherapy upfront does not mean any more or less treatment; it is just given in a different sequence. The most common way but to proceed with treatment of breast cancer is surgery following the diagnosis and if necessary chemotherapy followed by radiation, and then hormonal treatment. This is the most frequent order however the above are some common exceptions. For a better look at the chemotherapy flow chart below, be sure to check online:
http://BreastCancerHelpCenter.org/chemotherapy

CHEMOTHERAPY FLOW CHART

T   : Tumor Size

LN   : Lymph Node Involvement

ER/PR: ESTROGEN/PROGESTERONE RECEPTORS

Her2: Her2 Neu Receptor

+   : Present (Positive)

-     : Absent (Negative)

All obtained from pathology report

and used to determine need for

Chemotherapy

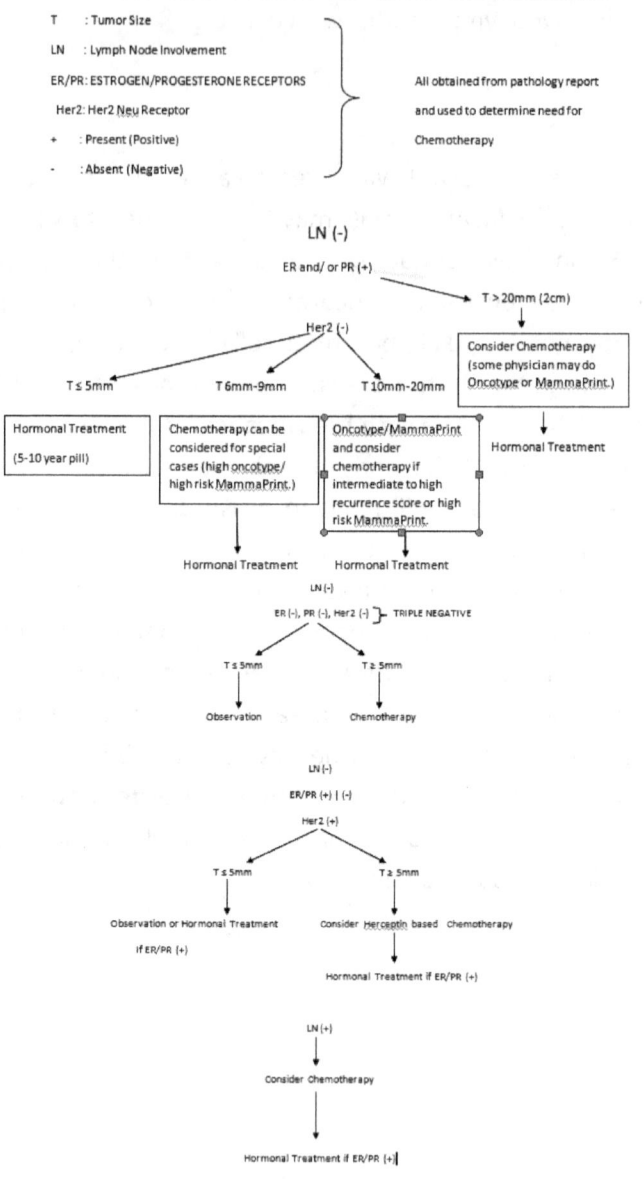

LN (-)

ER and/ or PR (+)

T > 20mm (2cm)

Consider Chemotherapy
(some physician may do
Oncotype or MammaPrint.)

Her2 (-)

T ≤ 5mm   T 6mm-9mm   T 10mm-20mm

Hormonal Treatment	Chemotherapy can be	Oncotype/MammaPrint
(5-10 year pill)	considered for special	and consider
	cases (high oncotype/	chemotherapy if
	high risk MammaPrint.)	intermediate to high
		recurrence score or high
		risk MammaPrint.

Hormonal Treatment

Hormonal Treatment   Hormonal Treatment

LN (-)

ER (-), PR (-), Her2 (-)] TRIPLE NEGATIVE

T ≤ 5mm   T ≥ 5mm

Observation   Chemotherapy

LN (-)

ER/PR (+) | (-)

Her2 (+)

T ≤ 5mm   T ≥ 5mm

Observation or Hormonal Treatment   Consider Herceptin based Chemotherapy

If ER/PR (+)

Hormonal Treatment if ER/PR (+)

LN (+)

Consider Chemotherapy

Hormonal Treatment if ER/PR (+)

This next section combines general guidelines and my personal opinion after treating breast cancer patients for many years. Please also refer to that chart which I have composed to accompany this section.

General Guidelines for Breast Cancer Treatment
» In general, patients with cancers which are lymph node negative and with an invasive component less than or equal to 5 mm in size do not require chemotherapy. That does not mean they will not need hormonal therapy or radiation but do not require chemotherapy.
» Patients with only duct cell carcinoma in situ do not require chemotherapy.
» Patients with pure tubular or Mucinous cancer do not need chemotherapy regardless of the size unless there is lymph node involvement which is very rare. Again, remember, some patients can have mixed cancers which are a different situation.
» Phyllodes tumors do not require any chemotherapy.
» If the cancer is lymph node negative and greater than 5mm in size chemotherapy may be considered in 2 scenarios: •If the cancer is estrogen and progesterone receptor negative or •HER2 positive

Let's look at this a little bit closer.

Remember, as I said before if the tumor is estrogen/progesterone receptor negative it is not under the influence of the female hormones and therefore will not respond to hormonal therapy. This is a more aggressive cancer! Again, estrogen and progesterone receptor negative cancers are much more aggressive. The only way we have to protect the rest of the body is with chemotherapy. The next scenario is the HER2 gene which if present defines an aggressive cancer. If the cancer is greater than 5 mm and has the HER2 gene then chemotherapy is needed. The difference is the chemotherapy cocktail must include the drug trastuzumab or Herceptin.

If there is lymph node involvement with cancer regardless of the estrogen/progesterone or HER2 status, the patient in my opinion chemotherapy needs chemotherapy. There are exceptions based on a person's age, illnesses and overall general health —meaning if someone is in a wheelchair has a bad heart and kidneys; no I am not going to give them chemotherapy. But if a patient is healthy and has lymph node involvement chemotherapy should be considered. There are some exceptions. If a patient has microscopic cancer in one of the lymph nodes (N1mic), a tumor less than 1 cm in size and is estrogen/progesterone positive, I might consider foregoing chemotherapy and just treating with hormonal therapy pills. This does not refer to patients with Immunohistochemical positive cells in the node, which we discussed above. This again is considered a negative lymph node. Other scenarios are:

Other Scenarios
» If the cancer is lymph nodes negative, greater than 2cm and estrogen/progesterone receptor positive, this is considered a stage two cancer and chemotherapy can be considered especially if the patient is premenopausal and healthy.
» Breast cancers with negative lymph nodes, 6-10mm in size and estrogen/progesterone receptor positive are in a gray area but most do not receive chemotherapy.

> » Cancers which are lymph node negative, estrogen/progesterone receptor positive, and between 1-2 cm. in size, will fall into a gray area with regards to chemotherapy and will frequently be tested with either an Oncotype or MammaPrint test –discussed below.

Some physicians will send a special test called an Oncotype to determine the aggressiveness of the cancer and if chemotherapy would be beneficial. Another option is a test called MammaPrint which examines the aggressiveness of the cancer. I am going to discuss this in more detail.

The Oncotype is a test performed by Genomic Health in California. It is used and approved only in cancers which are estrogen and/ or progesterone receptor positive and HER2 negative. In this test, a piece of the breast cancer from the surgery is sent to California and 21 different genes of the cancer are examined. Based on the results, a recurrence score between 1-100 is generated and divided into low, intermediate or high risk. If the recurrence score is between 0 and 17, the cancer is low risk - less aggressive with little benefit from chemotherapy. Intermediate risk is 18 to 31 and this tells us the cancer has some more aggressive tendencies and may benefit from chemotherapy but we really do not know. I tell patients that if they want to be aggressive then consider chemotherapy for intermediate recurrence scores but there is no right or wrong answers. There is a study called the Taylor RX trial which has been completed to determine the benefit of chemotherapy in the intermediate scores but the results are unavailable at this time. Recurrence scores of 32 or above are high risk which tells us the cancer is more aggressive and there is benefit from chemotherapy.

Another option is the MammaPrint test. In this test a piece of the breast cancer is sent to the company Agendia and a 70-gene analysis is performed. This will result in one of two results: low risk or high risk. There is no number associated with this test. Low risk cancers are less aggressive with less chance of spread. High risk cancers are more aggressive cancer with a higher risk of spread. MammaPrint does not predict the benefit of chemotherapy unlike Oncotype. Either of these tests is reasonable in the appropriate setting. It is important to keep in mind that neither of these tests take the size of the cancer into consideration. A 6cm tumor may have the same Oncotype score or MammaPrint risk as a 6mm tumor. However, a 6cm tumor in my opinion needs chemotherapy. So I only use these two tests if the results are going to change what I would do with regards to giving chemotherapy. Otherwise there is no need to order them. This is why I feel these tests are better used in the 1-2 cm size cancers which are lymph node negative, estrogen and/or progesterone receptor positive and HER2 Negative.

There are chemotherapy cocktails regimens which are used in early stage breast cancer. There are only a few drugs that are approved for treatment of early stage, meaning stage I, 2, or 3 breast cancer. Nearly every new drug developed for breast cancer is initially approved for stage 4. Hopefully with time it will work its way back to earlier stages but this can take many years if at all. Chemotherapy drugs which are used in early stage treatments are:

Early Stage Chemotherapy Drugs
» Doxorubicin (Adriamyacin)
» Epirubicin (Ellence)
» Cyclophosphamide (Cytoxan)
» Fluorouracil
» Paclitaxel (Taxol)

»	Docetaxel (Taxotere)
»	Methotrexate
»	Carboplatinum (Paraplatin)
»	Trastuzumab (Herceptin)

Drugs are used in various combinations based on clinical evidence and physician experience. These cocktails may be different depending on the characteristics of the tumor and the stage of the cancer. Some patients may only require 4 sessions of chemotherapy treatments while others may need more. Let's look at the most common combinations. The first section of combinations is the patients who are HER2 negative so there will be no trastuzumab (Herceptin) as part of the chemotherapy.

Treatment Protocols

Treatment Protocol	Notes
• A.C. doxorubicin + cyclophosphamide • Day 1: doxorubicin 60mg/m2. • Day 1: cyclophosphamide 600mg/m2. Repeat one time every 3 weeks for 4 cycles.	This treatment, commonly referred to as A.C. (Adriamyacin and Cytoxan), is given intravenously one time every three weeks for 4 treatments. It was a very common treatment used for many years until a slightly better regimen was approved. The regimen A.C. is still used but normally in combination with another drug (a taxane) administered after the four treatments. With all of the regimens you will see something called "M2" which is basically the way to calculate the drug dosage. It is based on the person's weight and height.
• T.C. docetaxel and cyclophosphamide • Day 1: docetaxel 75mg/m2 IV • Day 1: cyclophosphamide 600mg/m2 IV. Repeat one time every 3	This is given intravenously one time every three weeks for four cycles. This is the most common regimen used by itself now instead of A.C. It is generally used for stage1 or 2 breast cancers. Some physicians will give 6 cycles instead of four which I feel is okay

weeks for 4 cycles.	especially with stage 2 breast cancers. I use this regimen frequently.
• **A.C. (doxorubicin + cyclophosphamide) followed by weekly paclitaxel** • **Day 1: doxorubicin 60mg/m2 IV + cyclophosphamide 600mg/m2 IV. Repeat one time every 3 weeks for 4 cycles** • **After completion of A.C. above** • **Day 1: paclitaxel 80mg/m2 IV one time each week for 12 weeks.**	The A.C. is given in the traditional way one time every three weeks for four cycles and then paclitaxel is given intravenously one time every week for 12 weeks. This is also a common treatment especially in patients who have lymph node involvement or large cancers. I use this frequently.
• **A.C. (doxorubicin + cyclophosphamide) followed by paclitaxel** • **Day 1: doxorubicin 60mg/m2 IV + cyclophosphamide 600mg/m2 IV. Repeat one time every 3 weeks for 4 cycles.** • **After completion of AC above** • **Day 1: paclitaxel 175mg/m2 IV. Repeat one time every 3 weeks for 4 cycles.**	This is very similar to the prior treatment but if you notice on the diagram the paclitaxel is given as a much larger dose every three weeks instead of the lower dose weekly. This is the original way paclitaxel was given. It is still a very acceptable way to administer the drug. However a study (and I want to avoid studies in this book but I think this is important to understand this one) called ECOG1199 revealed it is better to deliver paclitaxel weekly as opposed to the larger dose every three weeks. There was an improvement in survival and also in my opinion it is easy to tolerate. I always use the weekly paclitaxel now following the A.C. when using these drugs together.
• **Dose-dense A.C. (doxorubicin + cyclophosphamide) followed by weekly paclitaxel** • **Day 1: doxorubicin 60mg/m2 IV + cyclophosphamide 600mg/m2 IV. Repeat one time every 2 weeks for 4 cycles.** • **After completion of A.C. above** • **Day 1: paclitaxel 80mg/m2 IV one time each week for 12 weeks.**	Notice in the prior treatments we have discussed, A.C. is given one time every three weeks for four cycles. In the dose dense protocol, A.C is given one time every two weeks for four cycles. This is again referred to as dose dense chemotherapy. This is a very confusing concept to understand. Cancers which are estrogen and progesterone negative are more aggressive and grow faster. The thought is by giving the treatments - A.C. closer together meaning every two weeks as opposed to every three weeks there is less time for recovery of some of the surviving cancer cells. It is still just 4 treatments. Cancers which are estrogen/progesterone receptor positive have no benefit in giving the chemotherapy every 2 versus 3 weeks. It makes no difference. It is tougher as patients on the every two week treatment plan do not have the extra week to recover from side effects. There is also a slight increased risk of blood transfusions in those receiving the treatment every two weeks.

• T.A.C. (docetaxel + doxorubicin + cyclophosphamide) • Day 1: doxorubicin 50mg/m2 IV, followed by cyclophosphamide 500mg/m2 IV, followed by docetaxel 75mg/m2 IV. Repeat one time every 3 weeks for 6 cycles.	This is commonly used for stage 2 and 3 breast cancers especially those with lymph node involvement. Some physicians prefer this regimen to A.C. followed by weekly paclitaxel and there is essentially no difference. Personally I find T.A.C. chemotherapy tough to tolerate and have also experienced more infectious complications. Nevertheless, it is still a very powerful treatment.
• F.A.C. (5-FU + doxorubicin + cyclophosphamide) • Days 1 and 8 OR Days 1 and 4: 5-FU 500mg/m2 IV. • Day 1: doxorubicin 50mg/m2 IV + cyclophosphamide 500mg/m2 IV. Repeat one time every 3 weeks for 6 sessions.	This is an older M.D. Anderson, Houston treatment but still used today. It is not used as frequently in the community but remains very acceptable for stage 1, 2, and 3 cancers. Sometimes it may also be followed by weekly paclitaxel for four weeks especially in cancers with extensive lymph node involvement.
• E.C. (epirubicin + cyclophosphamide) • Day 1: epirubicin 75mg/m2 IV + cyclophosphamide 600mg/m2 IV. Repeat one time every 3 weeks for 4 treatments/cycles.	This is not used very often. It's very similar to A.C. Adriamyacin and epirubicin are very similar drugs but epirubicin may be less toxic on the heart but is much more expensive.
• C.M.F (cyclophosphamide + methotrexate + 5-FU) • Days 1–14: cyclophosphamide 100mg/m2 orally. • Days 1 and 8: methotrexate 40mg/m2 IV + 5-FU 600mg/m2 IV. Repeat one time every 4 weeks times 6 cycles. OR; • Day 1: cyclophosphamide 600mg/m2 IV, methotrexate 40mg/m2 IV, and 5-FU 600mg/m2 IV. Repeat one time every 3 weeks for 6 sessions.	The C.M.F treatment has been a long standing treatment and is still used today. It can be administered as partially oral meaning using pills or IV. The oral administration of the drug cyclophosphamide is thought to be a little bit better but the IV formulation is easier and still acceptable. I have used this treatment in patients who are elderly or have other health issues but are still in need of treatment for their breast cancer. It is well tolerated for the most part and probably one of the few treatments that do not guarantee hair loss.
• A.C. (doxorubicin + cyclophosphamide) followed by docetaxel • Day 1: doxorubicin 60mg/m2 IV + cyclophosphamide 600mg/m2 IV. Repeat one time every 3 weeks for 4 cycles. • Subsequent cycles after completion of AC above. • Day 1: docetaxel 75-100mg/m2 IV once every 3 weeks for 4 cycles.	This was used commonly for many years and still is reasonable for lymph node involved cancer and higher stages. However, over the past few years many oncologists have started using the AC followed by weekly paclitaxel more. It is still a very acceptable treatment.

- T.C.H (docetaxel [Taxotere] + carboplatin [Paraplatin] + concurrent trastuzumab)
- Day 1: docetaxel 75mg/m2 IV, followed by carboplatin AUC 6. Repeat one time every 3 weeks for 6 cycles.
- Subsequent cycles
- trastuzumab 4mg/kg week 1, followed by trastuzumab 2mg/kg for 17 weeks, followed by trastuzumab 6mg/kg every 3 weeks to complete 1 year total of trastuzumab therapy. The first dose of trastuzumab start with the first day of docetaxel and carboplatinum. Another acceptable, more convenient approach is to deliver the trastuzumab every 3 weeks during chemotherapy as opposed to weekly.

The above treatments are only used for patients who are HER2 negative. Now let's look at some options for patients who are HER2 positive. The first treatment is T.C.H or docetaxel (Taxotere), carboplatin (Paraplatin) and trastuzumab (Herceptin). This treatment is given one time every three weeks for six cycles. Following completion of the 6 cycles the trastuzumab (Herceptin) must continue by itself to equal one full year of treatment. I do not want people to panic when they hear one full year of treatment because Herceptin itself does not give the typical side effects of chemotherapy. Herceptin is administered intravenously targeting the HER2 protein on the cancer cell so it spares some of the regular cells unlike chemotherapy which to be very honest is an atomic bomb that goes through and kills anything in its way and hopefully the cancer cells too. Patients who are receiving Herceptin alone frequently do not realize they are receiving the drug. Let's discuss some of the side effects later. Patients who are receiving this treatment will continue to overcome the side effects of the chemotherapy while still receiving the Herceptin. Radiation can start after the chemotherapy portion is finished as can hormonal therapy. You must think of Herceptin as targeted therapy not chemotherapy. T.C.H is my preferred treatment for HER2 positive patients.

- A.C. (doxorubicin [Adriamycin] + cyclophosphamide [Cytoxan]) followed by paclitaxel (Taxol) + concurrent trastuzumab (Herceptin).
- Day 1: doxorubicin 60mg/m2 IV + cyclophosphamide 600mg/m2 IV. Repeat cycle every 3 weeks for 4 cycles.
- Subsequent cycles
- Day 1: paclitaxel 80mg/m2 IV once time each week for 12 weeks, plus
- Day 1: trastuzumab 4mg/kg IV loading dose, followed by trastuzumab 2mg/kg IV once each week (or trastuzumab 6mg/kg IV once every 3 weeks) to complete 1 year of treatment.
  OR
- Cycles 1–4
- Day 1: doxorubicin 60mg/m2 IV + cyclophosphamide 600mg/m2 IV.

Another treatment option is adriamyacin and cytoxan every 3 weeks for 4 treatments followed by the weekly paclitaxel and trastuzumab (Herceptin). This is another popular way to deliver chemotherapy for HER2 positive cancers. However trastuzumab does not start until the adriamyacin and cytoxan portion is complete. This is because combining trastuzumab and adriamyacin together can cause an increase in heart complications. Frankly the particular type of HER2 based chemotherapy does really not matter. Some will say oncologists east of Mississippi tend to use more adriamyacin and cytoxan followed by paclitaxel and trastuzumab as this was tested by the NSABP Group in the Northeast of the U.S. Those west of the Mississippi tend to use more TCH as it was discovered by Dr. Slayman's team at UCLA. Whether this is true or not, who knows?

Repeat cycle every 3 weeks for 4 cycles.

- Subsequent cycles
- Day 1: paclitaxel 175mg/m2 IV. Repeat one time every 3 weeks for 4 cycles, plus
- Day 1: trastuzumab 4mg/kg IV loading dose, followed by trastuzumab 2mg/kg IV once each week (or trastuzumab 6mg/kg IV once every 3 weeks) to complete 1 year of treatment.

- Dose-dense A.C. (doxorubicin + cyclophosphamide) followed by dose dense paclitaxel + concurrent trastuzumab. - Day 1: doxorubicin 60mg/m2 IV + cyclophosphamide 600mg/m2 IV. Repeat one time every 2 weeks for 4 cycles. - Subsequent cycles - Day 1: paclitaxel 175mg/m2 IV one time every 2 weeks times 4 cycles. OR - Day 1: paclitaxel 80 mg/m2 IV one time each week for 12 weeks. plus - Day 1: trastuzumab 4mg/kg IV loading dose, followed by trastuzumab 2mg/kg IV once weekly until completion of paclitaxel. (or trastuzumab 6mg/kg IV once every 3 weeks) - Then administer trastuzumab 6mg/kg IV once every 3 weeks to complete 1 year of treatment.	This treatment is A.C. given in a dose dense fashion meaning one treatment every two weeks as opposed to every three weeks for four cycles followed by paclitaxel and trastuzumab. This is the dose dense way of giving chemotherapy with trastuzumab which again can be used in patients who are estrogen and progesterone receptor negative and HER2 positive. I do use this at times and patients seem to tolerate it well.
- docetaxel + concurrent trastuzumab followed by F.E.C. (5-fluorouracil [5-FU] + epirubicin [Ellence] + cyclophosphamide) Weeks 1–8 - Day 1: docetaxel 100mg/m2 IV. Repeat one time every 3 weeks for 3 cycles, plus - Day 1: trastuzumab 4mg/kg IV loading dose, followed by trastuzumab 2mg/kg IV once weekly for 8 weeks. - Subsequent cycles - Day 1: 5-FU 600mg/m2 IV + epirubicin 60mg/m2 IV +	This treatment combines the drug docetaxel and trastuzumab followed by F.E.C. I must admit I do not use the docetaxel at a 100mg/m2 as it is too toxic. However, it is a reasonable chemotherapy treatment based on European data.

cyclophosphamide 600mg/m2 IV.Repeat cycle one time every 3 weeks for 3 cycles.	

For more information on the treatment protocols, please refer online: http://BreastCancerHelpCenter.org/treatmentprotocols

Now we are nearly finished with the chemotherapy portion and I know you must be tired of all the medical jargon but I want you to think about some general principles.

I have not included every chemotherapy regimen for early stage breast cancer but 95% of the ones used are here. These will provide you with a good reference to use in speaking with your doctor. I want you to be familiar with the above regimens so nothing comes as a surprise when meeting with your oncologist. Most of these treatments can be used if necessary before surgery, the neoadjuvant setting, or after surgery, adjuvant. The next principle that I want to again reinforce is the purpose of chemotherapy, which is to decrease the likelihood of breast cancer returning to some other part of your body —lung, liver, and bone as well as distant lymph nodes being the most common places.

The next question patients will often ask is, "How do I know the chemotherapy is working?"

In the pre-operative or neoadjuvant setting when it is being given to decrease the size of the breast cancer, you can see the results in the breast. In the adjuvant or after surgery setting where chemotherapy is being given to cure any potential microscopic cancer cells that escape, you do not know if it is working. You pray the cancer never comes back. It is all about risk reduction. Please keep an open mind when discussing chemotherapy with your oncologists.

CHAPTER 7 - CHEMOTHERAPY SIDE EFFECTS

Chemotherapy side effects should be considered as inconvenient but manageable. Chemotherapy is there to do a job. It is designed to kill any remaining cancer cells that could be in the body. Please note that the side effects of chemotherapy pale in comparison to the return of breast cancer in a different part of the body. Cancer is the most dangerous poison that will ever attack your body. As we go through the side effects of chemotherapy, keep in mind that the various chemotherapy protocols will have different side effects.

Hair loss: This is likely the hardest side effect to deal with. Most early stage breast cancer treatments will cause it. The one treatment that may not is the CMF protocol. Hair loss tends to occur within about 14-17 days after the first treatment and always involves the hair of the head. Other body hair —eyelashes, eyebrows etc., has about a 50% chance of coming out. The hair usually starts to grow back within 2-3 months following completion of chemotherapy but that is variable.

Low white cells: White cells are one of the three main blood cells produced by the bone marrow. They fight infection and are important to health. Chemotherapy may lower the white cells and increase a person's susceptibility to infection. There are medications to counteract this. White cells are fast growing cells in the body and that is why they are affected by chemotherapy.

Infection: This is an oncologist's worst nightmare. This occurs normally, in the setting of the low white blood cells but not always. Many patients will have ports, which are IVs placed under the skin for chemotherapy, and these slightly increase the risk of infection It is very important that you notify your doctor, day or night, if you have a fever greater than 100.5 or hard chills, which may suggest you have an infection. Avoiding sick people is important but sometimes easier said than done. I ask patients to avoid raw food such as sushi, maintain good hygiene, and hand washing. The main thing is —just use common sense.

Nausea and Vomiting: This is a large concern for patients. Compared to several years ago, nausea and vomiting is not nearly the issue. Today, in my experience, up to 20% of patients may still have an issue or problem. Some chemotherapy protocols are more emetogenic (makes you sick) compared to others. There are many different medicines available to help prevent nausea. Some patients describe a low level of nausea that stays with them for weeks, frequently because of acid indigestion. Even though you may not think you have acid indigestion, the proton inhibitors such as Nexium, or Protonix may be helpful. Other useful ideas are to eat smaller meals, avoid constipation (nausea meds can cause constipation and constipation causes nausea) and also avoid spicy foods.

Constipation: Chemotherapy drugs can cause this, as well as the nausea medicines, especially a class called the 5HT3 inhibitors such as Zofran. It is important to drink plenty of fluids. I tell patients to drink at least 80 ounces a day. I also advise patients to take a stool softener for the first three days of treatment following chemotherapy. Again, constipation can cause all sorts of problems from nausea to bowel obstruction. If you go more than two days without a bowel movement, let your doctors know.

Diarrhea: This is another potential side effect but does not tend to happen as frequently with the regimens. If it does, Imodium A-D over the counter can be helpful. It is also very important to make sure that you remain adequately hydrated. If diarrhea continues for more than one to two days, let your physician know. The BRAT diet can also be helpful. This stands for bananas, rice, applesauce and toast. Basically, it means, avoid oily and spicy foods which may worsen diarrhea.

Joint Aches, Muscle Aches and **Flu-Type Symptoms**: These are quite common with breast cancer chemotherapy, especially with taxane drugs, docetaxel (Taxotere) and paclitaxel (Taxol). They may last a few days. Advil products can be helpful as well as good hydration.

Mouth sores: Mouth sores or mucositis, occurs at times when white cells are low. Now that we have ways to keep white cells higher, there aren't as many issues with mouth sores as before. A helpful prevention is to mix a quart of water with a pinch of salt and baking soda together, and gargle several times a day. If you do develop mouth sores, medicines are available. Good oral hygiene is extremely important.

Fluid Retention/Edema: We commonly see this with the drug docetaxel (Taxotere). It tends to worsen with increasing cycles of chemotherapy and heavy salt intake. The fluid retention is mainly in the feet, arms and face. Diuretics can be used but risk dehydrating someone. The fluid retention gets much better, six to eight weeks following completion of chemotherapy.

Taste changes and **Appetite**: The taste buds' changes are common and patients may have different cravings. During treatment, I tell patients not to be concerned about special diets because of taste changes —worry about appropriate dietary changes after chemotherapy. Patients tell me the only good thing about going through chemotherapy is they will lose weight. Well, this may not be the case as people can also gain weight. For the first few days following a chemotherapy treatment, patients may not feel well but then start to feel better and sometimes, carbohydrate-crave.

Menopause/Infertility: As discussed earlier, chemotherapy can cause damage to the ovaries and place a patient into menopause. Whether this is permanent or not, depends on many factors such as age, health and chemotherapy used. Many of the side effects that people attribute to chemotherapy are actually due to the hormonal imbalances as discussed before, such as hot flashes, depression/mood changes, joint aches and vaginal dryness. If a patient regains her period following chemotherapy, then pregnancy in the future may be an option. However, during chemotherapy it is important to use adequate birth control (not the pill) as pregnancy must be avoided.

Eye changes: Sometimes chemotherapy drugs can cause eye irritation or eye tearing. The lacrimal ducts just above the upper part of the nose, drain the eyes, and can develop scar tissue. This can cause the eyes to water almost like allergies. At times, lacrimal duct stents are required which will help the eye tearing. Also, prednisone eye drops may prove to be helpful but must be used with caution. The most common drug causing eye tearing issues is docetaxel (Taxotere).

Nail or **Skin Changes**: These are quite common with chemotherapy. Darkened lines across the nails may occur with treatment but eventually resolve with the nail growth. At times, patients may also get infections under the nail beds. Keeping the nails cut short and at times soaking them in warm water or apple cider vinegar can be helpful. Sometimes skin changes may occur such as darkening of the skin, and reddening of the palms and soles of the hands and feet. Chemotherapy can also sensitize someone to the sun, so it is important to avoid sun exposure without adequate protection.

Anemia or **Thrombocytopenia**: This concerns the lowering of red cells and platelets. These are the two other main cells produced by the bone marrow in addition to the white cells. Platelets prevent bleeding if you cut yourself, the red cells carry oxygen to various parts of the body. Platelets may decrease during chemotherapy but rarely to the degree where there is likely to be bleeding problems. Anemia or low red cells can occur frequently, especially with the dose dense protocols where the chemotherapy is given every two weeks instead of every three weeks. The risk of blood transfusions during traditional chemotherapy for early stage breast cancer is about 2%, and that number slightly increases with the dose-dense regimen.

Neuropathy: This is a common side effect with chemotherapy. The taxanes are mainly implicated in this side effect. Chemotherapy can attack some of the nerve in the hands and feet. This may cause tingling or numbness in the fingers and toes. This may worsen during treatment and continue for some time after. At times, the damage may be permanent but it usually gets better with time. Diabetics are more affected as they are prone to neuropathy. Sometimes patients may require a dose reduction in the chemotherapy. Medication such as B6 can be helpful. I also find glutamine powder helpful. Neuropathy may also result in walking and balancing issues. If the patient has pain with the neuropathy, medications are also available through physicians such as gabapentin (Neurontin) or Lyrica.

Cardiac or **Heart Side Effects**: The drugs doxorubicin, epirubicin and trastuzumab have heart issues as potential side effects. Normally, the issue with the heart is a decrease in the output, referred to as the ejection fraction of the heart which can lead to congestive heart failure. It is more common with certain doses of doxorubicin and epirubicin. If this occurs, the heart frequently returns to normal after cessation of the drugs. Epirubicin is thought to be a little safer than doxorubicin. The physician will usually perform an echocardiogram which is an ultrasound of the heart, or a MUGA scan, which is a more specialized x-ray to assess the heart prior to the use of these medications. Regimens with trastuzumab, which is less toxic to the heart, will be continued for one year so echocardiograms will be performed every few months.

Pulmonary or **Lung Toxicity**: This is an unusual side effect but can still happen, especially with the taxane drugs. The main lung issue is interstitial pneumonitis, where the lining of the lungs become inflamed. This can occur anytime and is treated with steroids. Also, with taxanes —mainly docetaxel, patients can get volume overload or edema, as we have discussed, which can cause breathing issues.

Leukemia: This is very rare but still a possibility. Leukemia tends to be more common with older drugs such as nitrogen mustard but can happen with any chemotherapy. This may occur many years later. The normal process of the patient is to develop a condition called myelodysplasia, which basically means bone marrow damage. Patients with myelodysplasia can progress to leukemia but many do not. This is also a risk for patients as they become older, regardless if they have ever received chemotherapy.

Chemotherapy Brain: Following chemotherapy, many patients experience a mental tiredness. They do not think as clearly, forget some basic words and have difficulty concentrating. This usually gets better with time but can linger. Some of these may be related to hormonal changes such as decreased estrogen, and, sometimes, it may be related to depression or anxiety.

Fatigue: This is a very common side effect. During chemotherapy, it is common to experience fatigue, which can be a cumulative process. People are more tired after the third cycle of chemotherapy compared to the first one. I advise patients to hydrate very well during chemotherapy and do some light exercise (walking or a mild jog if you are up to it) and get plenty of rest.

Allergic Reactions: Some medications are associated with allergic reactions which may occur within the first few minutes of treatment. It could be as simple as a rash or back pain, but can also be more serious, with low blood pressure, shortness of breath and, in very rare cases, anaphylaxis leading to death. If there are signs of a reaction, the chemotherapy will be stopped and a patient may be given steroids, intravenous fluids, oxygen, and antihistamines such as Benadryl or even epinephrine in severe cases. Patients tend to feel better very quickly. Doctors may ask you to take some steroids the day before and on the day of treatment to lower the likelihood of a chemotherapy reaction.

CHAPTER 8 - RADIATION THERAPY

Radiation therapy is an important part of your breast cancer treatment. Radiation is a local treatment meaning where they point the beam is where the effect is. This is unlike chemotherapy or hormonal therapy, which goes throughout the entire body. Radiation is basically x-ray beams designed to kill cancer cells. The treatment itself is painless and for the most part well tolerated. Radiation to other parts of the body can be tough but generally this is not the case for breast cancer patients.

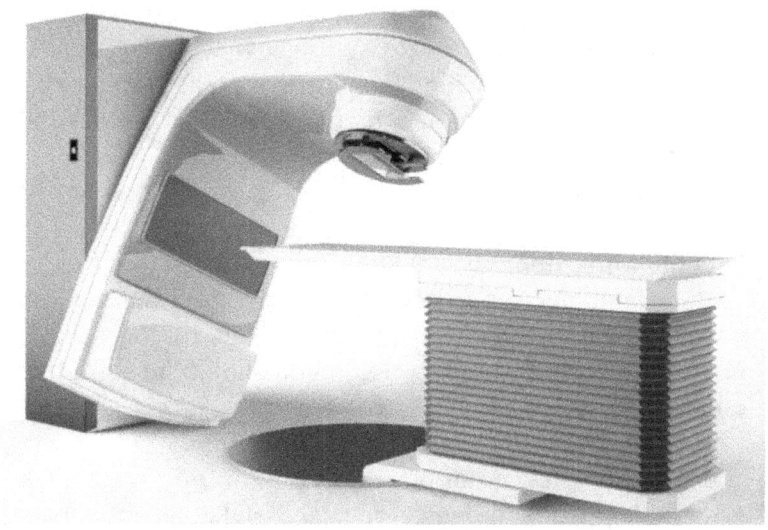

Who needs radiation?
» All patients who have invasive breast cancer and undergo lumpectomy, I have stated this before, if you undergo a lumpectomy from invasive breast cancer, you need radiation.
» Most patients who have DCIS or duct cell carcinoma in situ also

need radiation. There are a few exceptions and it is important to meet with a radiation oncologist.

» Patients who undergo mastectomy and have a tumor size greater than 5cm, 4 or more lymph nodes involved with cancer or very close (less than 1mm) or involved surgical margins also need radiation.

» Mastectomy patients who have 1-3 involved lymph nodes may also be considered for radiation. This is still controversial so meet with the radiation doctor.

» Patients who undergo neoadjuvant (pre-operative chemotherapy) for a large cancer, lymph node involvement or inflammatory breast cancer should also receive radiation following mastectomy regardless of how well they respond to chemotherapy. This means if there is a great response and no tumor is left at the time of surgery, radiation is still needed. The decision about radiation is based on the initial tumor characteristics.

» Patients with extensive lymphovascular invasion (see that section on the pathology report) or extranodal extension of the lymph nodes —meaning the cancer has broken through the lymph nodes into the surrounding tissue and should be considered for radiation.

» There is some new data that patients with triple negative breast cancers (estrogen, progesterone, and HER2 receptor negative) may also benefit from radiation even after mastectomy.

Types of Radiation

» **Chest wall radiation** which can be also done with reconstructed breasts. Whether or not the lymph nodes under your arms (axilla) or above your collarbone (supraclavicular) need to be involved with radiation will be decided by the radiation oncologist. Traditional radiation following mastectomy is normally a five-week process with radiation delivered each day.

» **Whole breast radiation** or **accelerated partial breast radiation** is done on patients who have undergone a lumpectomy. A uniform dose is given to the entire breast and towards the end of the radiation the x-ray is then concentrated on the incision site.

» **Accelerated breast radiation** or **Mammosite radiation** can be considered in patients who do not have extensive cancers. They have clear margins and a small breast cancer under 2cm. In this form of radiation a catheter with a balloon is placed into the tumor cavity by the breast surgeon. A radiation source is then placed into the catheter for a few minutes twice a day at least 6 hours apart. The program is for 5 days and then the radiation is complete. It is a quicker form of radiation and may be equivalent to the traditional whole breast radiation but long term follow-up comparisons are not available. If you consider this form of radiation you should question the surgeon or the radiation oncologist if you are a good candidate. Over the years I have seen many patients undergo Mammosite or accelerated partial breast radiation, many of which were not good candidates and the cosmetic outcomes were bad. It became very popular with breast surgeons because placing the catheter was very lucrative and still is lucrative. My tendency is to recommend whole breast radiation but mammosite can still be considered at times. Mammosite radiation is usually done before chemotherapy unlike traditional radiation which is done after completion of chemotherapy.

The side effects of radiation are usually well tolerated. The main side effects are fatigue, occasional radiation burns and a lot of inconvenience because of the Monday to Friday treatments for several weeks. However, most patients are in and out of the radiation center in ten to fifteen minutes. I find the side effects with mammosite more intense. There is also a possibility of breast shrinkage and contraction. Following radiations, patients also need to wait several months before proceeding with any type of reconstruction. Other side effects such as lung damage and heart complications are rarely seen with today's techniques. There are special shields to protect the vital organs from damage. There are some scenarios in which some patients should avoid radiation for breast cancer. One is pregnancy, another is prior radiation to the chest wall or breast, and another is connective tissue disease such as lupus or scleroderma. These patients tend have more toxicity.

CHAPTER 9 - HORMONAL THERAPY

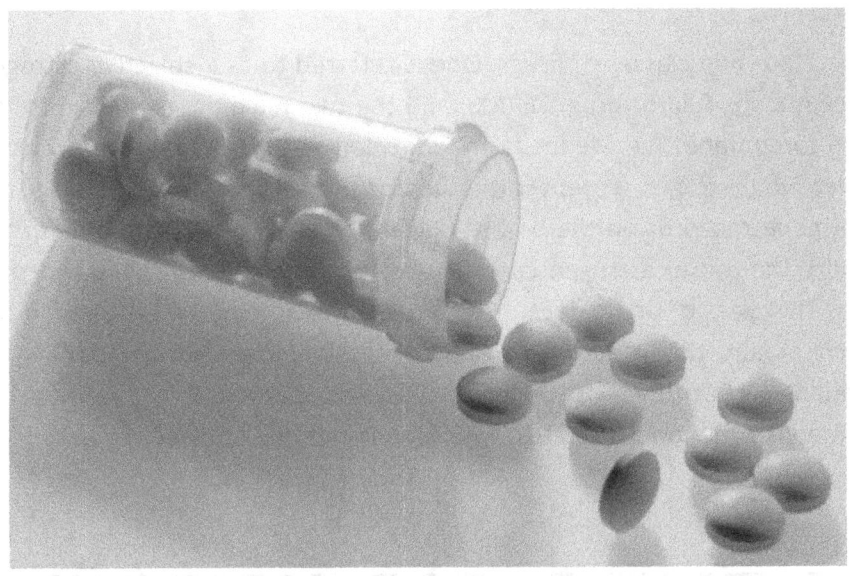

We refer to hormonal therapy as the treatment of breast cancer with pills which deprive the cancer of estrogen. Hormonal therapy in reality is anti-hormonal therapy. This is used in patients who are estrogen and/or progesterone receptor (ER/PR) positive and recall this is determined by the pathologist. All patients with invasive cancer, which is ER and/or PR positive, should receive anti-hormonal therapy. This is a very important part of breast cancer treatment. It is at least equal if not more important than chemotherapy. Like chemotherapy, hormonal therapy offers systemic benefit and is as powerful as chemotherapy without the side effects. It always amazes me that people go through chemotherapy, lose their hair, experience nausea etc. yet when I discuss the anti-hormonal pills with them they tell me, "no way have you seen the side effects of these medicines." It tells me the media paints a bad portrait of these drugs and by doing so, really does a big disservice to breast cancer patients. These pills are well tolerated and I would say, greater than 90% of patients have no problems.

There are two classes of drugs. One is referred to as a selective estrogen receptor modulator drug, SERMS, and the two main drugs are tamoxifen and toremifene. We will focus on tamoxifen as Toremifene is rarely used. Selective estrogen receptor modulator drugs work by blocking the hormone receptor on the breast cancer cell anywhere it could be in the body. Therefore, estrogen cannot feed the breast cancer cells and they die. This class of drugs does not decrease the amount of estrogen in the body. Again, this is a common misconception. **These drugs work in all patients, regardless of their menopausal status**. When we look at someone's menopause status, we divide it into one of three groups:

Menopause Status
» Premenopausal means they are still menstruating and have full ovarian function.
» Perimenopausal means they have stopped menstruating but still have some ovarian function and this can last for several years.
» Postmenopausal mean cessation of menses and no ovarian production of estrogen or removal of both ovaries —a bilateral oophorectomy.

Tamoxifen is the only drug used in someone who is premenopausal but also works in peri/postmenopausal women.

80

The other classes of anti-hormonal drugs are called aromatase inhibitors. The drugs in this class are anastrozole (Arimidex), letrozole (Femara), and exemestane (Aromasin). Aromatase inhibitors inhibit the production of the enzyme aromatase which is responsible for estrogen production. These drugs work only in patients who are fully postmenopausal. I have written a list of the generic and brand names of these drugs down.

Generic Name	Brand Name
Anastrozole	Arimidex
Exemestane	Aromasin
Letrozole	Femara

When someone is postmenopausal the ovaries are not functional or have been removed. This leaves roughly 10% of estrogen remaining in the body produced from the adrenal glands and fat cells. Remember how we discussed earlier that fat cells can produce estrogen and that is why it is important not to be overweight with breast cancer.

Aromatase inhibitors lower the remaining 10% estrogen of a postmenopausal woman to 1%. These drugs do not act at the cell level meaning they do not bind to anything on the breast cancer cells. Instead they reduce the amount of estrogen that is available to feed breast cancer cells. Patients who are pre or perimenopausal will be started on tamoxifen following chemotherapy. Tamoxifen is taken for 5-10 years and the major side effects are:

Tamoxifen's Major Side Effects
» blood clots (but no more than a birth control pill)
» uterine cancer (this is a small risk)
» hot flashes
» occasional vision changes

Studies did not prove that this drug causes weight gain, which is a misconception. Why do people feel they gain weight? Let's explore my theory behind this.

Frequently, patients who undergo chemotherapy are thrown into an early menopause. When people do go into menopause they have decreased circulating estrogen and their metabolism may change. So we can see occasionally weight gain as a result of this. The weight gain tends to coincide with, when they are starting tamoxifen. However, it is not related to the tamoxifen but instead, the change in metabolism which occurs from chemotherapy. Now, any drug can do anything so yes, some people could have some weight gain but studies suggest the majority do not.

As I said above, tamoxifen is normally taken for 5 years; however, results from the ATLAS study presented at the San Antonio Breast Cancer Symposium in 2012 stated that tamoxifen for 10 years is better than 5 years. This study revealed that those who took tamoxifen for 10 years had a 2.8% less chance of dying from breast cancer compared to patients who took tamoxifen for 5 years. This is not a huge number but in the fight against this terrible disease, I will take any percentage I can for my patients. There is a slight increased risk of death from endometrial or uterine cancer from 0.2% at 5 years to 0.4% at 10 yrs. There is also the slight increased risk of blood clots while continuing to take the tamoxifen. So what do we do with tamoxifen now in light of this new data? My approach is, if a patient has a small cancer which is lymph node negative, I will consider stopping the drug at 5 years. It also depends on the individual and how well they are tolerating the medicine. Each patient's input is essential. If the patient has a high risk cancer such as a large tumor or lymph node involvement I will keep them on tamoxifen for 10 years.

Another option is to change to an aromatase inhibitor if the patient has become postmenopausal. Remember, aromatase inhibitors only work in postmenopausal patients where tamoxifen works regardless of someone's menopausal status. Let's take a closer look at the aromatase inhibitors commonly referred to as AIs. I introduced this earlier. These drugs again are for fully postmenopausal patients. We can use tamoxifen also in postmenopausal patients but prefer to stay with the AI's as they are superior drugs in the treatment of breast cancer. The side effect profile I also feel is better. Now, like every drug, there is a list of side effects from here to kingdom come and patients may suffer side effects different to the ones I will mention. The main side effects seen with the AIs are:

Main Side Effects Seen With the AIs
» hot flashes
» joint and muscle aches(tend to get better with time if they do occur)
» mild bone loss

These drugs are also available now in generic form. At this time the AIs only have data that support for their use for 5 years. The first and still most commonly used AI is anastrozole (Arimidex), and this was proven to be better than tamoxifen in the big ATAC trial, which was Arimidex Tamoxifen Alone or in Combination. I try not to bore the readers with trials in this book but this an important one and I want to discuss it a little bit more. In this trial there were three arms. Clinical trials are like octopuses in that they have arms. This one had three. In one arm, patients receive Arimidex, in the other arm patients receive tamoxifen and, in the third arm, patients received both Arimidex and tamoxifen. It was found that patients who received Arimidex did better than those who received tamoxifen. Patients who received Arimidex did better than those who received the combination of Arimidex and tamoxifen. The combination of the two drugs was equal to tamoxifen. So something about combining these two drugs offset the benefit of receiving Arimidex. Based on this trial we knew that Arimidex was better than tamoxifen and also better than the combination of the two drugs —Arimidex and tamoxifen. Make sense?

Today, Arimidex combined with tamoxifen is not done as a result of this trial. However, if someone is not postmenopausal, we must use tamoxifen —there is no choice. The one important aspect of this trial is the fact that it has stood the test of time. All trials come out with claims, "greater than sliced bread" but the benefit of Arimidex over tamoxifen has maintained for many years.

I also want to look at the different ways of delivering hormonal therapy in general:

84

Ways of Delivering Hormonal Therapy

» The first is tamoxifen, which can be taken for five to ten years and, again, this is mainly for premenopausal patients or for patients who are unable to tolerate aromatase inhibitors.

» Next, any of the three aromatase inhibitors can be taken for 5 years but, again, only in postmenopausal patients (no exceptions).

» Another way to take tamoxifen is for 5 years and then letrozole (Femara) or anastrozole (Arimidex) for 5 years. This method has shown survival benefit in patients with lymph node involvement. But before starting letrozole or anastrozole, the patient must be postmenopausal.

» Another method is tamoxifen for 2-3 years, and then switch to an aromatase inhibitor for another 2-3 years, or even 5 years of the aromatase inhibitor. This is the switch method that has shown some benefit and used at times. Sometimes, I see this used in patients who are not fully postmenopausal and therefore start tamoxifen. Over time they become postmenopausal and we can switch to an AI. Why do we switch? Because we know the AIs are better than tamoxifen.

» Another less popular method but acceptable, is to start with the AI for 2-3 years and then change to tamoxifen to complete 5 years of treatment.

Now, let's discuss a little bit more about menopause and other things such as ovarian ablation. Menopause occurs naturally as a physiological change in a woman's life or after a surgical procedure when the ovaries are removed. If only the uterus is removed which we refer to as a total abdominal hysterectomy, it does not mean a lady is postmenopausal. Cessation of menses is not postmenopausal —only if the ovaries are removed. Another way a cancer patient can become postmenopausal is by going through chemotherapy. This is one of the ways that chemotherapy can be more helpful in premenopausal patients who are estrogen and/or progesterone receptor positive. With menopause, there is less hormones to feed any stray breast cancer cells. Chemotherapy can adversely affect the ovaries and place someone into menopause as we discussed earlier. When this occurs abruptly (as opposed to the slower natural process), the symptoms related to menopause including hot flashes, mood swings, and joint aches are initially worse. Sometimes a person may regain periods after stopping. However, with increasing age, this is less likely to happen. Even without periods, the person could be pre or perimenopausal for years.

So how can we determine if a lady is postmenopausal, when she is not having periods? Two blood tests are very helpful: Estradiol and FSH or Follicle Stimulating Hormone level. Estradiol is a measure of estrogen, and is low when the ovaries are no longer functioning. FSH is a hormone produced by the brain when it detects low estrogen. This hormone is trying to stimulate the ovaries to produce estrogen. Whether someone is postmenopausal, this hormone is constantly produced by the brain to stimulate the ovaries to produce estrogen but the ovaries no longer work. So, FSH is high and Estradiol is low when someone is postmenopausal. Anything in between is suspect that a person is not completely postmenopausal.

Another way to be made postmenopausal is a monthly injection given in the physician's office called, goserelin (Zoladex). This will shut down the ovarian production of estrogen. Some physicians will administer this injection to make sure a person is postmenopausal, and then prescribe the more powerful aromatase inhibitor drugs such as Arimidex or Femara instead of tamoxifen. However, at this time, there is no convincing data to support this. There are exceptions such as a premenopausal person who had a blood clot, and therefore, should not receive tamoxifen. In this case, we may need to make this patient postmenopausal, either by giving the injection (goserelin) or surgically removing the ovaries before prescribing an AI.

As we near the end of hormonal treatments, I want to discuss ductal carcinoma in situ and the use of hormonal treatment in this situation. Duct cell carcinoma in situ (DCIS) is an in situ cancer and there is no invasive component. Patients who undergo surgery for ductal carcinoma in situ are generally considered cured. We can however, use the drug of tamoxifen to decrease the risk of cancer coming back in the affected breast and also lower the risk of a new cancer in the opposite breast. Certain oncologists will recommend it based on a patient's individual circumstance. It is important to understand that the risk of DCIS spreading to another part in the body is only 1%. We have historically not used tamoxifen to decrease this risk because the side effects of tamoxifen potentially outweigh that benefit. If a patient has bilateral mastectomies, there is little benefit from tamoxifen. In addition, if the patient is estrogen and progesterone receptor negative, I have not used tamoxifen in DCIS patients. Please understand, the benefit of tamoxifen in DCIS is small but it is there.

As we conclude with the hormonal therapy section, I really want to emphasize how important this is with regards to breast cancer treatment. Please listen to your physician with an open mind and if this is recommended, it should be considered seriously.

CHAPTER 10 - SUPPORTIVE CARE

It is important to understand that chemotherapy treatments today are better tolerated. Many of the drugs used are the same but what has changed is the supportive treatment available to help people cope. Nausea and vomiting is not nearly an issue as it was before because of newer supportive medicines. There are different medications used to help prevent nausea. Some of these medications are given intravenously at the time of chemotherapy and include antacid medications as well as steroids. Steroids help prevent nausea and vomiting. There is also a class of drugs called 5HT3 inhibitors and these have been extremely beneficial in preventing nausea. You may know these drugs such as ondansetron (Zofran) or granisetron (Kytril). The longest acting drug is palonosetron (Aloxi), which lasts for 72 hours once given as an intravenous dose.

There is also a drug called aprepitant (Emend) that is available. This belongs to a class of drugs called substance P antagonist and it mediates its effect in the brain by blocking what we refer to as a neurokinin receptor. Again, it is not important to know these mechanisms, but what is important is that we know that this drug is frequently used in modern day chemotherapy. It has made a huge difference with nausea and vomiting prevention.

Another important supportive care treatment is a drug called Neulasta. Neulasta is an injection given the day after chemotherapy. It is mandated that we wait 24 hours following chemotherapy before this injection is administered. This drug increases white blood cells to lower the risk of infection. The white blood cells may still become low but they tend to recover faster, so the duration of infection risk is lower. In my opinion, this has made a huge difference in treating patients with chemotherapy. It has decreased the risk of infectious complications as well as mouth sores.

The sister drug of Neulasta is called Neupogen or G-CSF (granulocyte colony stimulating factor). However, Neupogen must be given as a daily injection for five to ten days unlike Neulasta, which is a one-time injection that has the equivalence of 5 to 10 days of Neupogen. This is an expensive shot but, in my opinion, well worth it. Not every chemotherapy regimen needs Neulasta. I use this frequently in my early stage breast cancer patients.

Medications are available to increase a patient's red cell count if they become anemic. We used this frequently in the past and you may have heard of these drugs —erythropoeitin (Procrit) or darbepoetin (Aranesp). However, it has been recommended that we avoid these drugs in patients with curable cancers. There was concern that these medicines may slightly increase the risk of return of the cancer. In breast cancer, there is no convincing evidence of this but, nevertheless, it is mandated that we avoid these drugs in patients with curable (stage 1, 2 and 3) breast cancers.

Modern day antibiotics to fight infections are very important. The days of using simple penicillin is long gone. We have very powerful medicines which are very effective. Frequently, if I see a sick patient, I have the ability to treat them in the cancer center with intravenous antibiotics and avoid hospitalization.

Some patients have said that Claritin may decrease some side effects such as joint aches or bone pain which can occur with chemotherapy and Neulasta. There is no scientific evidence to support this and I mention it because you will see it on the internet and it is a common discussion among patient groups. Another common side effect patients may have with Neulasta is back or chest pain, 7 to 10 days after chemotherapy. This is the body producing white cells which can be painful. There is a lot of bone marrow in the back and the breastbone of the chest.

Many cancer centers will offer classes as a resource for patients. This is where patients can meet with trained oncology nurses and discuss some of the concerns about their treatment as well review some of the side effects in more detail. This may be done as a group or on an individual basis. Please make sure you inquire if your cancer center has a chemotherapy class.

Another important supportive care treatment is a port (port-a-cath), which is a special IV that is placed in the chest wall and connected to the blood vessels in the neck. This makes it much safer and easier to deliver chemotherapy by avoiding constant IV placement. The nurses will put a numbing cream on the port and then place the needle into the port. There is a slight increase of infection with a port but overall, it really is beneficial and safer for patients. A PICC line is a special IV that can be placed in the arm. I prefer not to use this for breast cancer patients as it can limit the mobility of the arm and must be flushed daily.

Many patients inquire about holistic therapies and I think it is really reasonable to consider this as part of your treatment. Different forms of holistic therapy include taking vitamin supplements, massage, and different exercises. I feel strongly, that these can be helpful in coping with cancer treatment. However, these should not replace standard medical treatment. Alternative treatments used to replace standard therapies are not recommended. You should think very, very carefully before selecting alternative treatment as opposed to standard treatments.

CHAPTER 11 - GENETIC TESTING

About 7-10% of breast cancers are hereditary, meaning they develop because of a genetic mutation. The mutations are from the BRCA1 and BRCA2 genes. These are genes that belong to a class called tumor suppressor genes. When a patient has a mutation of one of these genes, there is an increased risk of ovarian and breast cancers. These mutations can be passed through generation. Situations in which these mutations should be considered in breast cancer patients are as follows:

Situations for Possible Mutations
» if a patient has bilateral breast cancer
» breast cancer before the age 50
» ovarian cancer at any age or a family history of ovarian cancer
» male breast cancer at any age
» Ashkenazi Jewish ancestry
» triple negative breast cancer under the age of 60
» family history of breast cancer in two first degree relatives
» greater than two family members with breast and/or pancreatic cancers

Patients with one of these mutations do have an increased risk of new breast cancers, or ovarian cancers. Mutations in men have an increased risk of pancreatic and prostate cancers. It should be noted that if a cancer develops as a result of the mutation, the prognosis is the same as someone who does not have a mutation but also develops a cancer. Having the mutation does not worsen outcome. It just increases the risk of new and different cancers.

Some options that can be considered if someone has a mutation:

Options to be Considered if Someone has a Mutation
» frequent imaging studies - mammograms or MRIs of the breast
» the surgical removal of both breasts and ovaries
» frequent gynecologic visits
» medicines such as oral contraceptive pills decreases ovarian cancer, but if you have breast cancer, you cannot use them.
» medicines such as tamoxifen or Evista can decrease the risk of development of breast cancer.

The tests to analyze the BRCA1 and BRCA2 mutation are expensive but frequently covered by insurance. The Health Information Privacy Act (HIPAA), prevents the use of these tests to determine insurance rates, eligibility or pre-existing conditions when considering insurance. Although 7 to 10% of breast cancers are hereditary (because of BRCA1 and BRCA2 mutations), there are also familial increases in breast cancer. This means, if you have a first degree relative (sister or mother) with breast cancer, you are at slightly increased risk of developing breast cancer. These patients do not have a definable mutation (that we know about at this time) but hereditary issues can play a role.

CHAPTER 12 - FOLLOW-UP

Finishing chemotherapy can be tough for patients. There are a few reasons to consider:

Why Finishing Chemotherapy is Tough for Patients
» Patients may feel abandoned as there are fewer office visits and not as much support.
» Patients feel they are not doing anything to prevent the cancer from returning after completion of chemotherapy and therefore, become scared.
» It is also common that patients will attribute every ache or pain to cancer. This is understandable and within the boundaries of human nature. Cancer professionals do the same because of what we see on a daily basis.

Upon completion of treatment, I see patients every one to two months to make sure they are coping and feeling better. If all is okay, we change the visit frequency to every three months for the first year and then, every six month visits unless there are issues or concerns. After five years, I will ask patients to come in once a year.

During follow-up visits, I do a complete physical exam and history and check blood work, including liver tests. Some cancer specialists will also check a blood test called a tumor marker. The tumor markers common in breast cancer are CA27.29 or CA15-3. These tests may be elevated if there is a return of breast cancer. The official recommendation by cancer organizations is that these tests need not be checked. This is because there are too many false positives —tests which are elevated with no evidence of cancer or false negatives— normal tests and there is cancer. However, many oncologists still check these and it is not wrong to do so. I am one of those who check them. If the patient feels well, the physical exam is normal and the tumor markers are normal, I feel better. Maybe this is more about my comfort level rather than the patient's.

Patients also ask about undergoing routine CAT scans, PET scans or bone scans. This is also very controversial and not recommended in the absence of symptoms. Let me explain why. If a patient has return of the cancer somewhere in the body, whether this is found by routine scan or waiting until the patient has symptoms, makes no difference with regards to survival. Once the cancer has spread, it is too late, it will not be cured. This again, is why it is important to be aggressive upfront. You will not get a second chance for a cure. Having said what I said about CAT scans, bone scans or PET scans, sometimes patients will tell me they just have more peace of mind undergoing a scan and I understand this completely. I will do whatever I can to help, with the understanding that it is not recommended to have routine imaging studies. It is always important to remember, you must call your doctor with unusual symptoms such as pain that does not get better, worsening shortness of breath or anything that is a concern.

CONCLUSION

As we finish this, I hope this has been helpful to you. I said before that this is by no means the most comprehensive book on breast cancer. A lot of what has been said is my personal opinion after years of treating breast cancer patients. I realize how tough it is to go through treatment. It is important to ask questions and listen carefully about your options. It is important to use this book as a rough guide as doctors may have slightly different approaches. If the approach is totally different from what is written here, consider seeking a second opinion. There are other forms of cancer which may affect the breast which are not discussed here. Remember, as you go through your fight with this terrible disease, you are not alone. There are many people who are also experiencing this. I wish you all the very best of luck. - Dr. Chris.

LINKS/RESOURCES

Websites
» http://BreastCancerHelpcenter.org/
» http://Cancer.org/

The American Joint Committee on Cancer (AJCC) has established staging by the TNM method.

TNM definitions

Primary tumor (T):

TX: Primary tumor cannot be assessed T0: No evidence of primary tumor Tis: Carcinoma in situ; intraductal carcinoma, lobular carcinoma in situ, or Paget's disease of the nipple with no associated tumor.

Note: Paget's disease associated with a tumor is classified according to the size of the tumor.

Paget's Classification of Tumor Size
» T1: Tumor 2.0 cm or less in greatest dimension
» T1mic: Microinvasion 0.1 cm or less in greatest dimension
» T1a: Tumor more than 0.1 but not more than 0.5 cm in greatest

dimension

» T1b: Tumor more than 0.5 cm but not more than 1.0 cm in greatest dimension

» T1c: Tumor more than 1.0 cm but not more than 2.0 cm in greatest dimension

» T2: Tumor more than 2.0 cm but not more than 5.0 cm in greatest dimension T3: Tumor more than 5.0 cm in greatest dimension T4: Tumor of any size with direct extension to (a) chest wall or (b) skin, only as described below.

Note: Chest wall includes ribs, intercostal muscles, and serratus anterior muscle but not pectoral muscle.

» T4a: Extension to chest wall

» T4b: Edema (including peaud'orange) or ulceration of the skin of the breast or satellite skin nodules confined to the same breast

» T4c: Both of the above (T4a and T4b)

» T4d: Inflammatory carcinoma*

*Note: Inflammatory carcinoma is a clinicopathologic entity characterized by diffused brawny induration of the skin of the breast with an erysipeloid edge, usually without an underlying palpable mass.1Radiologically there may be a detectable mass and characteristic thickening of the skin over the breast. This clinical presentation is due to tumor embolization of dermal lymphatics with engorgement of superficial capillaries.

Regional Lymph Nodes (N)

» NX: Regional lymph nodes cannot be assessed (e.g., previously removed)

» N0: No regional lymph node metastasis.

» N1: Metastasis to movable ipsilateral axillary lymph node(s).

» N2: Metastasis to ipsilateral axillary lymph node(s) fixed to each other or to other structures.

» N3: Metastasis to ipsilateral internal mammary lymph node(s).

Pathologic Classification (pN)

» pNX: Regional lymph nodes cannot be assessed (not removed for pathologic study or previously removed)

» pN0: No regional lymph node metastasis

» pN1: Metastasis to movable ipsilateral axillary lymph node(s)

» pN1a: Only micrometastasis (none larger than 0.2 cm)

» pN1b: Metastasis to lymph node(s), any larger than 0.2 cm

» pN1bi: Metastasis in 1 to 3 lymph nodes, any more than 0.2 cm and all less than 2.0 cm in greatest dimension

» pN1bii: Metastasis to 4 or more lymph nodes, any more than 0.2 cm and all less than 2.0 cm in greatest dimension

» pN1biii: Extension of tumor beyond the capsule of a lymph node metastasis less than 2.0 cm in greatest dimension

» pN1biv: Metastasis to a lymph node 2.0 cm or more in greatest dimension

» pN2: Metastasis to ipsilateral axillary lymph node(s) fixed to each other or to other structures

» pN3: Metastasis to ipsilateral internal mammary lymph node(s).

Distant Metastasis (M)

» MX: Presence of distant metastasis cannot be assessed

» M0: No distant metastasis

» M1: Distant metastasis present (includes metastasis to ipsilateral supraclavicular lymph nodes).

AJCC stage groupings
» **Stage 0**   •Tis, N0, M0
» **Stage I**   •T1,* N0, M0
» **Stage IIA**   •T0, N1, M0 T1,* N1, ** M0 T2, N0, M0   •*T1 includes T1mic ** The prognosis of patients with pN1a disease is similar to that of patients with pN0 disease
» **Stage IIB**   •T2, N1, M0   •T3, N0, M0
» **Stage IIIA**   •T0, N2, M0 T1,* N2, M0 T2, N2, M0 T3, N1, M0 T3, N2, M0   •*T1 includes T1mic
» **Stage IIIB**   •T4, Any N, M0   •Any T, N3, M0
» **Stage IV**   •Any T, Any N, M1

Recommended Reading

In my quest to better my understanding on how to help patients deal with the sudden news of having breast cancer, coping with medications, surviving through therapy, patiently adhering to follow up sessions and eventually outlasting this tribulation. I found these books to be helpful and recommend them to all who would need help in matters related to breast cancer. You can check them out on my site here:

http://BreastCancerHelpcenter.org/recommended

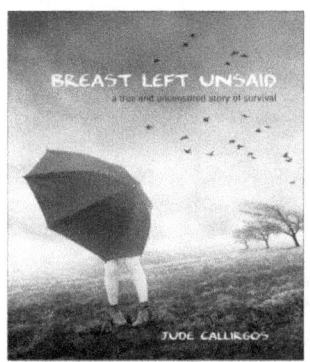

Breast Left Unsaid

A genuine story of survival wherein one woman triumphs over the stages of hurricane-like circumstances that occur in her life; divorce, death of a loved one, seriously ill parents and the sudden news of having breast cancer.

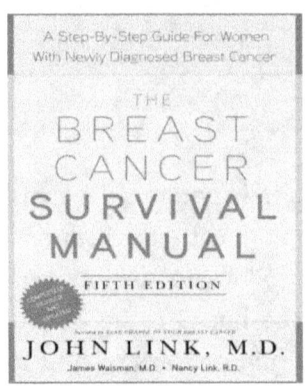

The Breast Cancer Survival Manual

The leading cause of death in women from 35 to 54 years of age, breast cancer is one of the most terrifying and confusing diseases ever. This book contains the latest findings to help women face treatment, feel informed and empowered.

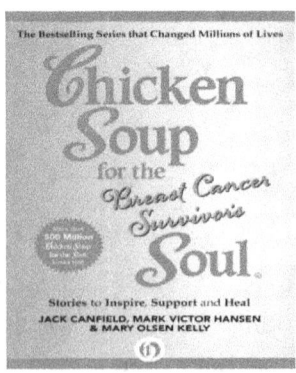

Chicken Soup for the Breast Cancer Survivor's Soul

Find hope and strength in the inspiring stories of how family members and victims face their fears in what could be their darkest hour. This book showcases the human spirit and how it shines through even when confronted by something as uncertain as breast cancer.

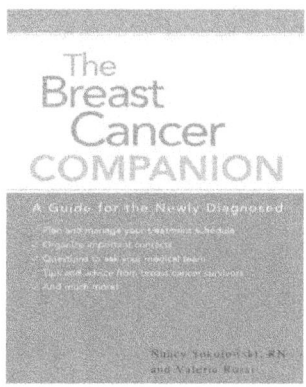

The Breast Cancer Companion

This book provides a vivid step-by-step process for those going through breast cancer. For the families, relatives and loved ones concerned, you will find plenty of useful insight and information. For breast cancer victims, solace and comfort in your silent breast cancer companion.

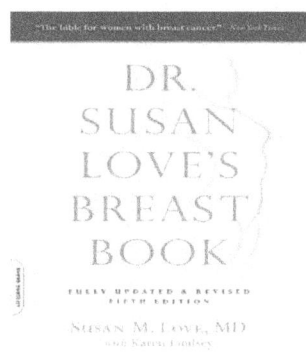

Dr. Susan Love's Breast Book

The long standing "bible" for the newly diagnosed with breast cancer, this book provides a full blown guide not just for patients, but for all who are interested in knowing the decisions, treatment and other concerns related to this disease.

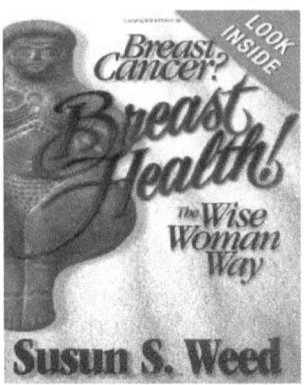

Breast Cancer? Breast Health! The Wise Woman Way (Wise Woman Herbal Series)

For those who want to remain "breast cancer free" or to those who have recently been diagnosed with one, this book offers a lot of information with how to keep up and go on living a full and happy life.

About The Author

Dr. Chris was born in Europe but has lived in the US for many years. He attended college both in Europe and the US and completed medical school at the University of Texas. Residency and fellowship in oncology was completed at Baylor.

Dr. Chris has spent many years taking care of cancer patients with a strong emphasis on breast cancer. He has been very involved in clinical research serving as the lead investigator on several important trials in breast cancer research and treatment. He continues to be very active in research serving on numerous committees and panels devoted to breast cancer. Dr. Chris has also authored and co-authored articles on breast cancer which have been published in prestigious journals and presented at national meetings.

Dr. Chris remains very committed to research and helping eradicate this terrible disease. The education of his patients and the community also remains a top priority.

Dr. Chris resides with his family and enjoys reading, traveling, and movies. He is excited to share the Breast Cancer Help Center with you.

You can find Dr. Chris on Google+ and Facebook.